Printed in the United States of America

First printing 2014

ISBN: 9781496112644

AMAZON PUBLISHING

www.amazon.com

FOREWORD

I first met John in my office in Roseville, CA. He had been referred by Sunrise Natural Foods here. He informed me the Oncologist had done the surgery under his left arm, to remove some of the 26 tumors seen in the P.E.T. scan, Melanomas in the lymph system. His doctor painted a dark picture of his future, namely that he would not live longer than six months. I then obtained his blood readings and, based on those results, his immune system was low and he was near death.

My job as an HNT (Health Nutrition Therapist) is to recommend a protocol or plan of natural substances and supplements to rebuild a healthy immune system, which I did in John's case. He also informed me that he refused chemotherapy, radiation, and interferon as treatment modalities. His doctor would not discuss any natural remedies and even told him he has never studied other alternatives. John felt angry and very disappointed in his M.D.s attitude and lack of knowledge. John then began taking an essential amino acid supplement and suggested antioxidants, including many different remedies, addressing his kidney and liver dysfunctions. Gradually over many months his strength showed signs of improvements. It was a real battle for the past four years to maintain his focus on eating correct foods and avoid foods which might cause toxicity in the blood and body systems.

Having been a Biology major in college and having studied organic and inorganic chemistry, John began to research the latest possible remedies for his own cancer and, over the past two years, possible alternative remedies for other types of cancers. I notice he is diligent in his approach, objective as possible, and has discovered many different plants and supplements which could stop some cancers in their tracks. John has become a believer in the science of natural foods as a preventive and most of these, he feels, far surpass those chemicals made in the labs as a challenge to cancer cells. John learned these chemists spend hours in the laboratories of our universities and pharmaceutical buildings to create expensive drugs which will be sold at ridiculously high prices. They even mix known nutritional plants which allay cancer, or mix them with chemicals in order to enlarge the profits for their companies.

But for John the proof is now in natural foods and supplements, which are what the body demands to stay healthy. On the other hand, when modern day synthetic drugs are imposed on the body, it rebels, revolts and gets sicker from the foreign products manufactured as a synthetic. The body just knows intuitively what it needs for its health.

It is now well documented by science when the body is fed vegetable and fruits, it assimilates them comfortably and with no harmful side effects. It digests better, does not rebel, and feels good as it becomes stronger and healthier. Again, the opposite is true of synthetic chemicals, which more often than not, creates immune deficiencies and lowers the body's resistance to disease—particularly on the subject of cancer. The body accommodates well to the fruits and veggies (especially the dark greens), and to the leaves and barks of the tropical areas which are made into supplements.

John also emphasizes when it comes to conquering cancers, the truth is in our blood. Man-made chemicals are not smarter that God's creations. In summary, John is convinced we don't always need a double-blind study to prove the efficacy and effectiveness of our good eating habits. In his case, eating the correct foods helped heal his body from the attacking melanomas, built its own defense army, and blocked cancers pathways to form cancer tumors. It is clear to me, if John had not followed my recommended protocol he would not be with us today to provide this book for those fighting cancer.

It has been four years now that John has been my patient. Through his own cooperation and some of his own research, he won the battle over cancer, is healthy, vibrant, and full of life daily. We Holistic doctors don't use the language that a patient is in remission: John's cancer is gone. His blood results demonstrate his body is in charge of his life, not melanomas. John's first book "Beating Cancer Can Be Fun—Cancer fighting Strategies for first time diagnosed patients" set the process in motion to educate those recently diagnosed. The process of keeping the body alkalized, eating the best foods, and avoiding harmful foods works for most cancer patients. This book broadens and expands knowledge for all cancer patients, not just for the first time diagnosed patients.

My own opinion is you should read this book and others suggested by John. Read them with care. It is your body and you can make the best choices for it. Stay focused and do what you think will work. Have a Holistic doctor guiding your path to recovery. Still consult your own M.D., always be asking for his opinion in not only what may prolong your life with minimal suffering, but also the odds for a total cure of your condition.

I personally wish all you readers of this book for a happy trip and, most of all, for the positive results you seek for your life.

--by Dr. Ward Joiner, DC, HNT Roseville, CA

ACKNOWLEDGEMENTS

To my Chosen One, Dr. Ward Joiner, DC, HNT who from the beginning five years ago provided me with hope, inspiration and the right nutritional protocol which saved my life.

To Alden Okie, sales consultant at Sunrise Natural Foods in Roseville, CA, who guided my path just after the surgery, by referring me to Dr. Joiner.

To all the medical Nutritionist Doctors who provided the research and information and advice so that my body could heal from a deadly Melanoma in the lymph. I salute you all.

To Brandy Gilmore, red cell Nutritionist, who goes above and beyond her training in the blood cell analysis, with words of support to encourage me to press on, not give up in seeking out the nutrients necessary for my body to heal. You are truly one of the miracles in my healing process.

To my sons and daughters who gave a positive listening ear when I chose the Holistic path to recovery. Many thanks and much appreciated.

To Dominique Javier, who edited and performed the arrangement of photos, paragraphs, and some sentences in the completion process of this book. Thanks!

To David Mock of No. Carolina, who was my best computer technical assistant when he lived in California. My computer was hacked and phished, but he helped me save the bulk of chapters and we put them in "the cloud."

Lastly, thanks to the Amazon Company for creating this space so that I could send this invaluable data on eBooks.

TABLE OF CONTENTS
YOU CAN HEAL YOUR CANCER

CH 27 Is There a God, Holy Spirit, or Higher Power Protecting Me?

PREFACE

KILLING CANCERS THE NATURAL WAY

This is my testimonial: as a cancer survivor of over three and a half years, my extensive research of which nutritional and water supplements aided me throughout my recovery process. As I mentioned in my first book BEATING CANCER CAN BE FUN, my Oncologist and a veteran Oncologist-Urologist stated that most likely I would not survive as "there is no known cures for Melanoma." In fact I discovered the cancer that is least written about and least researched is Melanoma in the lymph system. Within a week of my surgery, I located Dr. Ward Joiner, DC, HNT and hired him as my Holistic doctor. Thank God I learned early on that medical doctors in private practice limit themselves in the treatment of cancers in what is becoming an outdated mode of therapy for those with chronic conditions. Yet, Holistic doctors expand their knowledge of how to make the immune system healthy with nutrition and supplements and other modalities which help the cancer patient heal.

Compared to my first book, I have broadened my information to include the best breakthrough discoveries by M.D. researchers who specialize in nutritional cures for stopping cancer spread and, in many cases, actually cure cancers once and for all. You won't read Allopathic writings which go outside the narrow scope of chemo and radiation. Some conventional researchers are beginning to see that, perhaps, mixing natural foods with chemo makes the sickening poisons less poisonous and enables the patient to suffer less. But as far as curing cancers, conventional professionals still live in the dream world of trying to kill cancers with chemicals manufactured in the laboratories of America and elsewhere. It has become evident the goal in medicine, generally speaking, is to manufacture remedies which are very costly and will make them and pharmaceutical companies big money. It is clear to me they don't always operate in the best of interests of those with phase III and phase IV cancers for sure. What good does it do if you invent a chemical mixture that costs the patient and their insurance company $5,000 or $10,000 per treatment, which slows cancer progression, but still isn't a cure?

I also discovered that patients are forced to see Holistic or Naturopaths when their cancers are out of control because the conventional doctors have given up on them—and are advising them "to get their affairs in order." My big question is why doesn't the medical profession wake up and recommend (not prescribe) a nutritional schedule to help the patient build strength so that the immune system can adequately defend itself against the free radical avengers? Many doctors are aware that their own peer M.D.s who have done the nutritional research have made amazing discoveries in the past 20-30 years, yet they look the other way and continue using chemical formulas to kill cancers which don't work. It is sad to think the cancer patients are being rendered such a gross disservice, and are dying by the hundreds of thousands due to this avoidance of other alternatives than the conventional ones. After all, the conventional ones used today, of chemo and radiation, have not affected the survival rates of patients for fifty years and, in fact, the statistics show patients are dying at a faster rate than fifty years ago.

And so now you, the reader, know my motivation for writing this second book:

1) To share the recent discoveries with nutrients from the earth and ocean.

2) To share my own testimonial and that of other cancer survivors.

3) To remind you the cancer industry is in trouble by not expanding their methods of research. Note: The NCI does invest in some "alternatives" for just a small amount of money. They allot most of it to the largest and their favorite hospitals for "research." However the monies are spread so thin to the grantees, there is little hope any positive results will occur.

4) To be sure to detoxify your body to assure the nutrients are absorbed in your system.

5) To provide a list of foods to eat, and foods to avoid.

6) To emphasize the importance of drinking alkalized water and maintaining an alkalized medium in our bodies.

7) To provide a list of professionals who you can research and learn from, to advance your knowledge of the prevention and cures for cancer.

8) To highlight the relevance and importance of adopting a psychological and spiritual perspective when diagnosed with cancer.

9) To encourage you to self-research and learn all you can about your potential for complete cancer recovery and to utilize the services of a veteran Holistic doctor, as well as your chosen Allopathic M.D.

By JOHN W HALL, AUTHOR, MA, MFT

www.authorjohnhall.net

916-705-6624

CH 1

DEDICATED TO THOSE WHO HAVE A CANCER DIAGNOSIS, REGARDLESS IF IT IS PHASE I, II, III OR IV

Have you been told by your doctor your cancer is one of the most dangerous kinds of cancer and immediate action is needed? That you must be rushed into chemo, radiation or surgery? That there are no other choices for you, or the doctor?

But wait a minute! If some folks are being cured by other methods, why is the whole truth being withheld from you? I was cured of chronic Melanoma in the lymph glands without chemo poisons, radiation burnings; however, I did have surgery to remove part of the metastasized cells. No interferon either as my doctor said it wouldn't improve anything and might cause suffering. In addition, there is plenty of documentation of cancer patients who recovered from their cancers with the use of corrected nutrition under the direction of a skilled Holistic doctor, just as I was cured by a healthy Nutrition plan by Dr. Ward Joiner, DC, HNT. I want to emphasize here Dr. Joiner treats the Immune System, not cancers per se. The body can then gather its soldiers and fight and destroy the cancers.

Today, five years later, I am perfectly healthy again, in spite of what I had been told after my surgery that my odds of survival were unlikely. Melanoma is one of the fastest moving cancers, particularly when it enters the lymph system and spreads throughout the body. By adapting the nutritional protocol from Dr. Joiner, I am fortunate to be alive today. I can do aerobic exercises, ride my bike longer distances, and swim in the pool at my workout gym.

MAIN PURPOSE OF THIS BOOK

This book is dedicated to all cancer patients who want to explore other systems of treatment before they might move forward into surgery or one of the traditional treatments. My desire is to offer you more than just words of hope, but rather to empower you to become not hopeless victims of the disease, but be fully in charge of the best possibility with which to treat your cancer for recovery. It was with such empowerment that I was able to select a Holistic professional and eventually conquer my cancer. And I might add, it was fun to have chosen a winning formula!

There is one pre-condition I ask of you before I share lifesaving information. And it is this: If you believe cancer will kill you, it probably will. On the other hand, if you believe in the guidance of a Holistic doctor coach, then you are stating you might be able to conquer your cancers. Thus, you have changed your mind. It is not impossible. Medical doctors will lead many of you to believe that death is inevitable and refuse to even refer you to a trained HNT. Those doctors have a narrow focus and tend to operate within the 9 dots of their reality. As expert transformational leaders will say: they, to become transformed, need to learn to think and research outside the 9 dots. Perhaps then they will be able to claim to cure cancers.

Above all, be open to change. Be open to the fact that traditional medicine methods of choice are quite limited. And it is your life, so you don't have to limit yourself to whatever remedies you find. M.D.s are limited to 3 methods: chemo, radiation or surgery. Most doctors did not study a focused course in herbs, plants and natural supplements in medical school. And only a few educated themselves afterwards. Worst of all, their focus is not studying the immune system; thus, they don't comprehend its importance in healing cancer. In fact, most of them will not discuss nutritional remedies with you in their offices. Fact is in some states, it is illegal for them to discuss alternative options with you. They are experts in describing to you the progression and phases of illness, but not to discuss the progressive stages of healing—so the body can rebuild its natural strength to fend off and destroy cancer cells.

The focus here is to provide you with updated information and research on cancer prevention by skilled medical researchers, from books, articles, the internet, and from the results cancer patients have attained with the use of alternative sources. All of this leading to the healing of different parts of the immune system in order to heal the body. It is well documented and my belief the body's system of cells, organs, tissues and blood vessels are designed by nature to heal itself and protect us from invasion by pathogens, viruses, bacteria, and fungi. And so far the only true solution is to correct the elements or foods we put into our bodies. Does anything else really work?

Clearly then I write this book to you, the patient, for the following reasons:

1. To learn a clear vision towards your nutritional health.
2. To provide the means to avoid or eliminate the pangs, misery and doubts that Allopathic doctors cast you into.
3. To learn the statistical odds for recovery or death by entering into traditional treatments vs. holistic treatments.
4. To provide basic suggestions for a diet designed to strengthen the immune system.
5. Data on how to keep the body alkalized with certain foods and waters.
6. To encourage you to have supportive people around you during your process of recovery.
7. To demonstrate the destructive elements of medical professionals, including the Pharmaceutical companies, the non-research doctors, and the less educated nurses—especially in teaching nutritional methods to address cancers.
8. To cite examples of where the FDA is being helpful or hurtful in relation to effective cancer treatments.
9. To learn the psychological and spiritual aspects of recovery and how they do make a difference toward your recovery.
10. Suggestions on how to overcome your fears and doubts, to be able to grasp a sense of being in order to have a peace and understanding of your predicament with your cancer.

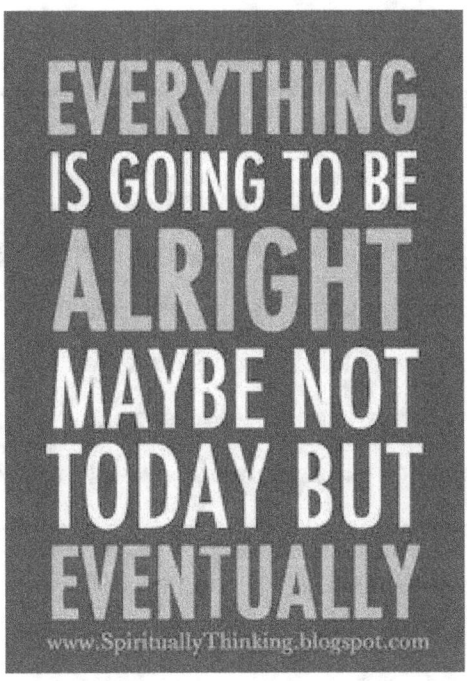

EVERYTHING IS GOING TO BE ALRIGHT MAYBE NOT TODAY BUT EVENTUALLY

www.SpirituallyThinking.blogspot.com

CH 2

PERFECT HEALTH - A REAL POSSIBILITY

My main goal in confronting my cancer when it was first diagnosed was DON'T QUIT YET (if ever). No matter what you have been told by anyone, your doctor, friends, relatives, etc., it is most likely not true. Most people have not done their homework and have only piecemeal data on the subject of how one might survive from the disease. Ask anyone to explain a good definition of the immune system. Odds are they can't. Most physicians can't either. Perhaps M.D. researchers who are on top of their game can explain it the best. It is a complex network of blood and lymph in the organs, blood vessels, and blood systems. It contains all the necessary nutrients to keep us alive and healthy. It is nature operating within our bodies.

So the question arises, can we attain perfect health if we eat well on a regular basis? Is our daily diet reliable to fight off the free radicals leading up to cancer, the invading enemy? When our mothers told us when we were kids to eat our vegetables and fruits on a regular basis, did we believe it and follow her directions? Was she fully aware of foods to avoid and what is best for us? Did anyone ever alert us to the fact that Coca-Cola and Pepsi cola have absolutely no food value and, in fact, have such an overload of sugars that they, coupled with other sugar foods, could be contributing to our diabetes, heart issues, and lead to cancer someday?

Did the schools, or anyone, inform us of how the large farms in America are genetically modifying our foods, lessening our ability to assimilate enough vitamins and minerals in order to sustain our healthy bodies and avoid becoming sick? Were we sufficiently warned of the dangers of cigarette smoke, dangers in chemical companies, radiation from many newer inventions, toxins which were placed in the walls of many of our schools, i.e. asbestos materials?

A STEPPING STONE TO THE FUTURE OF THE SEARCH FOR PERFECT HEALTH: THE "WHAT IF" EXERCISE TO ORIENT THE MIND TOWARDS POSSIBILITY THINKING

What if you knew of a way to stop cancer spreading? What if you knew of a way to stop cancers from forming tumors? What if you found out that foreign chemicals that enter the body actually hinder the health of normal cells? What if you discovered cancers cannot live in a highly oxygenated environment? What if you learned cancers feed off and grow faster in an acidic body? What if you met some M.D.s that specialize in slowing and stopping cancers with solely natural foods and supplements? What if they could show you how to beat your cancer with dark greens and fruits, with no side effects? What if you learn some of the best antioxidants are from the weeds in the ocean?

What if you learn chemo poisons injected into a cancer patient actually can cause cancer to spread? And that radiation to the patient will create a high acid state in the body, which might encourage the growth of cancer cells? And what if the medical profession awakens, after 50 years and billions of dollars into research projects, that chemo and radiation, in the majority of cases, had not cured cancers? The evidence is surfacing in this regard - 500,000 plus patients will die of cancer this year alone.

What if you learned pharmaceutical companies solicit and groom medical students, while they are studying to become M.D.s, so that they sort of "own them"? They wine and dine them, give favors, and set them up to use their laboratory manufactured chemicals after they graduate. The doctor today is controlled by the propaganda the pharm companies advertise to the public, so that patients later on will dictate to doctors which meds they want (even if they don't work). In other words, what if some pharmacies are giving bonuses to doctors, to prescribe their products to unknowing patients?

What if you discovered that the oxygen so vital to healthy cells, is the real core issue in defeating cancer? That oxygen deprivation in tissue actually is a major issue in a cause of cancer development? That there are natural remedies to correct malfunctioning cells which become cancerous?

So the question again: IS PERFECT HEALTH POSSIBLE? My impression and that of Nutritional Research physicians, is a definitive

"YES". I suggest you read some of the research of doctors working with the Life Extension program. Their research and conclusions are optimistic, mostly accurate, and certainly are major contributions to cancer patients who want to live longer, and with minimal or no suffering.

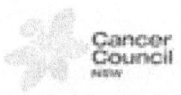

CH 3

HOW COGNITIVE DISTORTIONS CAN PREVENT THE BODY'S HEALING

(at the end of this chapter, questions to ask your M.D. doctor before possible surgery or radiation or chemo)

As a trained Family Therapist, many of the people I have counseled distort the truth about themselves, others, and events they have misunderstood. Some might label these negative thoughts as opposed to positive thoughts. It's almost like some of us get fixated on their negative thoughts which makes one feel weaker in the body and in brain function. Studies have revealed the immune system does weaken with angry thoughts, heavy judgmental thoughts of others, heavy sadness over time, depression, and heavy worry and anxiety.

Here listed are some negative thoughts which might prevent growth of the immune system:

1. My doctor says "herbs are dangerous to your health." Of course this would cause an extreme worry and anxiousness in the individual. So how do I overcome this mental-emotional state? First by doing your own check list and gaining new information about whatever herbs. Try researching the Wikipedia Encyclopedia on the Internet. They will provide you with a ton of information and names of herbs for healing the body.

2. Second, you might self-sentence to yourself: "I can't (won't) face my cancer." To this I say yes you can. Dealing with fear of this type is not new on the planet. That feeling of helplessness and hopelessness usually hits all of us who have been diagnosed with cancer. We have probably heard from various sources that cancer kills. However, let's look at the facts. If we believe cancer cells are smarter than us, perhaps we are going to be eaten by them. However if we can figure out how to beat them, then we might overcome them. To gain control over the situation psychologically, physically and spiritually is the challenge. In particular we want to get beyond our heavy fears. I have been there, done that—so I know it can be done. And you don't need a college degree or be a talented scientist to explore in all these areas. The fact that you are reading this book is definitely a head start.

3. Third, my doctor said "don't deal with those quacks", as if he is an expert in quackery. Clearly he distrusts Holistic doctors who sell and promote supplements from their offices in the past. Some Holistics may have been corrupt in their dealings with people. Yet how many M.D.s are corrupt when 187,000 people a year died in hospitals last year by medical treatments which killed them? So let's face it: there are some good physicians and some bad too. The

goal then for me was to search for a talented Holistic Doctor like Dr. Ward Joiner, DC, HNT who could recommend foods and supplements that heal.

4. Fourth, doctors often imply that you are a Phase III or IV. So what? So they have become experts in predicting stages of cancer progression. Yet the bulk of them are ignorant, lacking knowledge to lead to a cure for cancers in most cases. They have chosen to follow an Allopathic or a conventional way of treating cancer with only chemo poisons, radiation burnings, and surgery. A very narrow minded mental set. In reality, how do they know what Holistic doctors do for patients when they themselves haven't even studied which healthy foods and waters will help a cancer patient get well? M.D.s rarely took any courses on Nutritional health in medical schools.

My key question to the medical profession is: Why aren't you designing a schema to show the progression of rebuilding the immune system, so that our own body can repel and fight the cancer cells invaders? A Phase I through IV? We cancer patients are only interested in recovery and not the pessimistic Phase I-IV of medical folks. We want physicians to get on a track of saying to us: "Little by little you are getting better. Your immune functions show improvement now."

5. Fifth, do you remember the key words Tony Robbins and top corporate trainers implement when he teaches dynamic leadership? YES WE CAN. YES WE CAN. YES WE CAN! This is a necessary philosophical position for those of us with cancer. We can overcome. It will take effort. It will require a support team of professionals and relatives and having positive people in our lives during our crisis. Yes we can do some things differently in our

lives. Yes it will require a concentrated effort on our part. No it is not always easy, however I can say: In my case it was worth it. And it can end up to be fun when you begin winning the game.

Here I want to share an experiment done by Dr. Masuru Emoto which blew my mind, but it convinced me more than ever of the power of the mind for all of us:

Through the 1990s, Dr. Emoto performed a series of experiments observing the physical effects of word, prayers, and music on the crystalline structure of water. He hired photographers to take pictures of water to the different variables and then they were subsequently frozen so they would form crystalline structures. The results were nothing short of remarkable. The shape of a crystal where negative words were said, such as "I will kill you", shatters the picture of it. When positive words were said, such as "I love you", the entire crystal shone brightly and gave a beautifully formed hexagonal photo. Many physicians have observed where family members prayed over a cancer relative, he got well and overcame symptoms. The Power of the Mind sends out energy and is powerful force. Certainly it wasn't just the prayers which accelerated recovery, but a change in lifestyle and eating habits too.

According to Dr. Emoto, "slang words will totally destroy the structure of water." He added that the intention of the speaker or what is written near the water will have a significant result on the structure of the water. The word "anger" totally destroyed the crystal structure. He feels the water consciousness senses the intent of the person.

If thoughts can do that to water, I can imagine what they can do to us— especially since we are 60% water. Emoto says water has memory and we affect how we think, giving off vibrations. And vibrations are resonant energy. For example, if we know "smoking kills" then we are giving off a negative energy—and, ergo, this is not healthy for the human body.

In summary, Dr. Emoto discovered that crystals formed in frozen water reveal changes when specific, concentrated thoughts are directed towards them. He found the water that came from clear springs shows brilliant, complex and colorful snowflake patterns. In contrast, polluted waters exposed to negative thought forms were incomplete, asymmetrical patterns with dull colors.

To view the photos of the different crystals, go to www.highextistence.com/water-experiment. Truly remarkable that our thoughts have such power in the universe, both individual thoughts and intentions and group mind intentions!

QUESTIONS TO ASK YOUR M.D. WHEN FIRST DIAGNOSED

1. What evidence do you have that chemo or radiation work? What are short and long term effects of surgery in my case? If you were diagnosed with cancer like mine, what would you do?

2. Specifically what chemicals will be placed in my body if a surgery is done? What food preparations should I eat before and after a chemo treatment, to offset undesirable symptoms?

3. If neither chemo nor radiation is recommended, do you have any experience with using alternative methods, such as nutrition, supplements, acupuncture?

4. What are the death statistics given this sort of surgery? Survival rates?

5. If the doctor says he has no experience with Nutritional protocols, ask him for a referral to a Holistic physician.

6. Ask him if he gets cancer, will he permit the use of chemo or radiation?

7. Ask how urgent it is to have the surgery done immediately, or can I wait another month or two to decide?

8. Ask how many surgeries has he/she personally done? Successes or not?

9. Predictable after effects and recovery rate after the surgery?

10. Does he do any follow up if the patient becomes a Phase III or IV, or does he just abandon him and let him go home and die?

WE CANCER PATIENTS DESERVE TO KNOW ALL THE PARTICULAR INFORMATION ABOUT OUT DIAGNOSIS, PRIOR TO ALLOWING A DOCTOR TO DO SURGERY, DO CHEMO OR RADIATION, OR ANY OTHER PROCESS. IF HE FAILS TO COOPERATE AND ANSWER QUESTIONS FULLY, YOU HAVE THE WRONG DOCTOR. THE SAME WITH A HOLISTIC PRACTITIONER: IF HE AVOIDS OR TRIES TO RUSH YOUR DECISION BEFORE RECOMMENDING A SPECIFIC PROTOCOL, YOU BEST SEEK OUT A SECOND OPINION. THE MAIN QUESTION TO ASK: WHAT ARE THE SIDE EFFECTS OF A PARTICULAR FOOD OR SUPPLEMENT? WHAT RESULTS CAN BE EXPECTED FROM THE DATA?

CH 4

INTEGRATIVE MEDICINE VS CONVENTIONAL MEDICINE

It is important to understand the terms or definitions used in the discussion of cancer treatments. The terms complementary and alternative medicine are often used interchangeably. However, they are two different approaches to the treatment of disease. The following terms portray the meanings of the different therapies:

Conventional medicine, or "Traditional" medicine, is practiced by a medical doctor (M.D.), a doctor of Osteopathy (D.O.), and other allied health professionals. Other terms used are: Allopathic, western, and biomedicine.

Alternative medicine consists of therapeutic approaches used in place of conventional medicine. Integrative medicine combines traditional, western and complimentary approaches, but does not replace conventional therapy. It may be used for:

*Managing symptoms

*Increasing wellness or quality of life

*Improving treatment outcomes

Note: these are terms as defined by the MD Anderson Cancer Treatment Center.

So the question arises: Is integrative therapy right for me, such as acupuncture, yoga, and nutritional supplements? Anderson Center insists there should be clinical and scientific evidence to support their use. Many patients report the successful use of complimentary uses, others had no positive effects.

Anderson states before trying any complimentary or integrative therapy, it is important to consider:

*Safety (appropriateness of your condition, quality control of herbal medicines or supplements)

*Effectiveness

*Cost in time and money

*Credentials of the practitioner

As an answer to the question: What complimentary/integrative treatments are recommended for cancer? MD Anderson does not make any recommendations. However they do have a bias, they do assist patients and doctors in deciding what types of therapies might be integrated into conventional cancer treatment (i.e. chemotherapy and radioactive). This seems to directly contradict their original statement that they make no recommendations for complimentary/integrative therapies. They state their intent is to require evidence-based reviews of complimentary therapies, including research studies published in medical journals. They admit some, but not all, of these results show effectiveness; and for that reason, these therapies are not recommended without first consulting your physician. The poor patient is unfortunately left in the dark and this conclusion to consult with one's physician is, in most instances, meaningless. Why? Because most Oncologists have only a minimal knowledge of herbs and plants and effective antioxidants. And many more have no updated knowledge of their efficacy. In my case, my 56 year old Oncologist who did my surgery admitted to me: "I just do cutting. I know nothing about nutrition, nor can I refer you to anyone in town who can assist you." I was informed I would die soon. Fortunately, I knew how effective antioxidants can be, and Dr. Joiner convinced me that I needed to "energy up" my immune system--and then the body would know how to heal itself when fed correctly. It worked and, five years later, my blood test shows no more signs of Melanomas in the lymph system! Of course I learned in my own research that the conventional use of chemo (poisons) and radiation actually lower the immune system. Ergo, they are not safe, cause suffering, and are not even effective in most cases (with only few exceptions). My conclusion: if MD Anderson used the same criteria for the treatment of cancer for the Allopathic or conventional treatments, utilizing chemo and radiation, they should logically ban their usage in general.

They speak to the Naturopaths about that they must demonstrate how effective their products, using the language EVIDENCE-BASED PROOF. Using the same logic, if we insist the Allopathic or conventional doctors need to show EVIDENCE-BASED PROOF that chemo and radiation are wonderfully effective, we have the answer. Statistics show they are basically ineffective, with only a few exceptions. The side effects of both are cruel, tortuous, punishing, and blatantly should be barred by the FDC. And they don't even come close supporting the immune system - which IS the only way cancer can be stopped in 95% of the cases.

CH 5

CANCER ORIGINS—WHERE CANCERS ORIGINATE

Most of us cancer patients want to know how to trace the origins of their cancer. We may know it already, or we may never find out with any certainty where it came from. In my own case, my Melanoma originated when I exposed myself to intense sun rays over many summers as a young person, without any sun screens. I have since learned I furthered my own causations by too much sugar intake with candies, ice cream, cookies, pastries, and chocolate milk. All of them created a high acidity in my body and cancers grow faster in such an environment. Presently I only go out in the sun before 9 a.m. and after 5 p.m. for about 10 minutes—using sun screen ointments for sure.

In the list below I am sure I was exposed to many of these factors as well. Hopefully you will learn from this list some of your own possible causative factors:

*Food contaminants in dairy and meats

*in City, County and well systems (waters high in acid content)

*in GMOs (genetically modified organisms) placed in our crops or foods

*in cigarettes (see FDA warnings)

*in acid based waters, minerals

*in food packaging, processed foods

*in microwaves, there is a loss of vitamins in the foods placed inside

*in plastic bottles (a leakage of chemicals)

*In amalgams placed in teeth (Mercury poisoning)

*in certain poisonous fuels

*in smoggy air (from factories and freeways)

*Sun exposure to skin

*in old contaminated building, schools, homes, especially asbestos infected

*chemo poisons used by medical professionals to treat tumors, cancers

*pH imbalances of either too much Alkaline or too much Acid content in blood

*Sewage dumps-give off soil and air contaminants

*hospital deaths from chemicals (an estimated 187,000 patient deaths last year in the U.S.

*Nature's pollution (trees, plants, forest pathogens and fungi)

*House cleaning chemicals

There are many more causative factors leading to cancers. I forgot to mention that I have had 5 root canal surgeries and, in each case, had amalgams removed which had Mercury with the silver. I recall that for years I had a severe viral attack each winter. After my 3rd removal, I simply don't get viruses anymore.

It is important to emphasize IT IS YOUR JOB TO TRACE THE CAUSES OF YOUR OWN CANCER, if at all possible. Admittedly, I was surprised how many causes there were to my accruing Melanoma.

When I go shopping today, sucrose content and sugar content in the foods are always a focus. Let me share some of my experiences in the store:

Bottled sodas usually have 28 grams of sugar, candy bars have high content unless it is marked dark chocolate with a no sugar or low sugar marking. Incidentally dark chocolates are o.k. if you have cancer. Most packaged foods are loaded with high sugar content. I buy no sugar syrup instead of the high sugars in maple syrup, or the maple syrup artificial type. When you buy yogurt watch out for high sugar marks because you can buy just plain yogurt. Fruits have a lot of sugar content, so it is recommended by Holistic doctors to not consume them in large quantities. Ask your Doctor about this one. Coca Cola and Pepsi and their products are high sugar and must be avoided. I personally drink diet Pepsi in low quantities. What about bakery goods in the bakery section? For the most part, I avoid all their products because the sugar contents are not even marked on most of their foods. Usually you can tell they are high in sugar by just looking, as the sweets are coated with brown and white sugars.

Since I reduced my sugar intake, I feel much better and am more mentally alert. And the fact that my cancer has not returned warms my soul even more. And I did get a big bonus as in the past two years – I lost 20 pounds due to decrease in sugars, carbohydrates, and white bakery goods.

CH 6

PROTOCOLS WORKING TO KILL CANCER

Dr. James Lowenstein, M.D. uses a combination of different herbs or natural substances to help patients overcome their cancers. In an article reprinted from www.newswithviews.com, he shares his potent information and product:

All immune suppressive diseases are associated with an increased rate of malignant diseases including lymphoma, leukemia, and Hodgkin's disease. Patients who are immune suppressed from chemotherapy drugs and radiation develop Kaposi's sarcoma, non-Hodgkin's lymphoma, cervical cancer and Hodgkin's disease. Organ transplant patients and patients with autoimmune diseases have an increased incidence of cancer because of the use of immune suppressing drugs. The reason is the immune system is involved in recognizing and destroying cancer cells.

THE LIFE ONE PROTOCOL

Several natural substances have been proven of value in treating cancer and HIV:

*Chrysin: a flavenoid derived from Passion Flower with antioxidant properties, increases Tumor Necrosis Factor, binds estrogen receptors, and inhibits HIV action.

*Criolus Versicolor: a Chinese mushroom with antioxidant effects, stimulates the immune system, inhibits invasion of cancer cells metastasis, and has antiviral activity.

* Dinololy methane: a phytochemical found in cruciferous vegetables (broccoli and brussel sprouts), inhibits the adhesiveness, movement and ability to invade cancer cells, and has anti-estrogen effects on cancer cells.

*Resveratrol: is a non-flavenoid phenol found in grapes which is an antioxidant, prevents platelet clumping, blocks resistance to insulin, inhibits abnormal estrogen, and blocks viral replication in HIV

*Tumeric extract (Circumin): a potent antioxidant, inhibits insulin resistance, inhibits metastasis, and has beneficial effects in HIV viral reproduction.

*Quercertin: a flavenoid that brings out programmed death of cancer cells (apoptosis), an antioxidant and anti-inflammatory, and reduces cholesterol and LDL values.

*Green Tea extract: contains epigallocatechin chemical which is a primary anti-cancer agent.

*L-Selenium Methionine: an antioxidant stimulates the immune system and helps restore Selenium which is low in cancer patients and HIV patients.

*plus the Protocol contains a Liposomal matrix

According to Dr. Lowenstein, Life One cures a variety of cancer types: breast cancer, colon cancer, prostate cancer, cervical and ovarian cancers and acute promyelocytic leukemia. Clinical trials are quicker when done with patients who have not done chemotherapy or radiation. Life One has 2 U.S. patents as an immune enhancing product. Clinical trials were done in patients with malignancies in Mexico and Venezuela.

Dr. Lowenstein is a Board Certified specialist in Internal medicine who cared for office and hospital patients for 34 years; then 4 years of research into natural substances convinced him natural plants are safer and more effective than most conventional chemicals, and generally less expensive than pharmaceutical drugs.

His research culminated in writing the book: A Physician's Guide to Natural Health Products that Work. He can be reached via his book. The Doctor lives outside the U.S. in Costa Rica so that he can use safe and effective treatments which the FDA would not likely support. He claims a high rate of cancer recoveries and says that rates can be improved by addressing:

    *eating a low glycemic diet

    *healing endocrine damage with DeAromatase

    *correcting hormonal imbalances (usually estrogen excess)

    *finding and eradicating bacterial infections in non-responding patients

    *diagnosing and treating fungal infections

    *correcting deficiency of adrenal and testosterone hormones in advanced cases

    *preventing narcotic use which stimulates the growth of malignant cells

In the bulk of all my own researches, there are only two doctors who are as complete and knowledgeable and thorough with immune deprived cancer patients: Dr. Ward Joiner, DC, HNT and Dr. James Lowenstein, MD. My own protocol that I used to get well has many similar recommendations as Dr. Lowenstein.

But there are several approaches I utilized which he does not mention:

1. Constant measurement of the pH level and drinking alkalized water. Recall a heavy acid content in a cancer patient is not healthy, since cancers thrive from acid mediums and die in alkaline or basic mediums.

2. Use of the live red blood cell tests under microscope to determine which nutrients the body is lacking. It is also a more certain way to track the patient's progress in terms of their use of corrected foods. In my own case I lacked B12 vitamins, had insufficient water intake, and excess sugars in my system.

3. Dr. Joiner recommends the top quality supplements over the months of treatment—since all manufacturing of vitamin, mineral and herbal companies are not the same quality. He knows the difference and so the patient can depend upon having the very best quality supplement intake. The same advantage for patients with these two docs is easy access by long distance phone calling. They take the necessary time to coach and educate the patients—which most conventional doctors won't take the time, nor do they have the knowledge with which they can suggest possible cures for the malignancies. As a local California doctor, it is easy to have direct access for patients within the U.S. www.myholistic health.net – Dr. Joiner's site. I must remind the reader: Dr. Joiner does not treat cancer per se, instead he insists he helps the patient power up their immune system so that the body's natural functions will ward off the cancers. He recommends many of the protocols which Dr. Lowenstein utilizes for his patients.

Again to contact Dr. Ward Joiner, HNT, DC in Roseville, CA, call 916-791-5555.

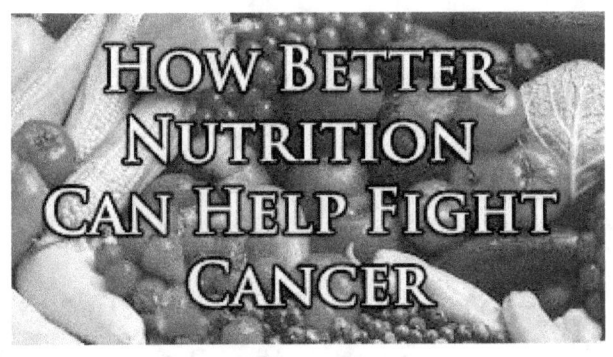

CH 7

RECENT BREAKTHROUGHS WITH ALTERNATIVE
NATURAL SUPPLEMENTS

I discovered some of these through Jenny Thompson's HSI site on the internet. These are exciting! I use some of them, others not yet. My cancer is now totally arrested and my CAT scan is negative to any cancers. Nonetheless, I want to list each one in this chapter for your immediate viewing. I suggest, if one or two of them might apply in your own cancer, you speak with a knowledgeable Holistic or Naturopathic doctor for his recommendation.

Some of this may be highly technical information with chemical terminology that is difficult for you. Try to get used to hearing and familiarizing yourself with some of the terms used. Why? Because they may serve you well and save your life.

The six ingredients I will expand upon here came from the wonderful research done by the Health Science Institutes medical staff (HSI). A booklet titled "Today's Greatest Alternative Medicines, pp. 19-31, with some of my own comments intermixed with their observations:

1. HSI PANELISTS WITH SEAWEED CANCER TREATMENT

"It's a weed and a slimy weed at that. But unlike the ones that invade your lawn, this weed might actually do you some good. It has been cited as a primary cause for record-low cancer rates in Okinawa, Japan. It was used—with reported success—to treat and prevent radiation sickness following the Chernobyl meltdown in Russia. It has yet to be tested in a human clinical trial. But according to panelist Kohhei Makise, M.D., the Japanese medical community is being inundated with reports as to how this medicinal seaweed has helped thousands of Japanese patients fight cancers."

Dr. Makise recently wrote us in a long, extended email discussing several new natural remedies that are producing successful results among his patients. But in this report, we decided to focus on a natural immune builder that is so new to North America that we'd never heard of it before.

It's called Fucoidan, a complex of polysaccharides (carbohydrates) found in brown seaweed, mostly found in Asia-Pacific variety known as Kombu. The seaweed has been a dietary staple in Japan since the second century B.C. And in Okinawa—which posts Japan's highest rate of Kombu consumption—it has reported produced considerable health benefits. And the residents there enjoy some of the longest life spans in Japan and the single lowest cancer rates in the country.

SEAWEED EXTRACT CAUSES CANCER CELLS TO SELF-DESTRUCT

In the 1990s, scientists identified Fucoidan as the primary immune-building substances in brown seaweed and began to test it. In one case, they injected female lab rats with a carcinogen known to produce mammary tumors. They fed half of the rats a standard diet, then fed the other half a standard diet and added daily helpings of brown seaweed containing fucoidan, and monitored the animals for 26 weeks. The fucoidan conveyed two substantial results: First, the fucoidan fed rats developed fewer tumors than the control fed rats. 65% developed breast cancer, 76% in the control rats. Second, the fucoidan fed rats resisted developing tumors for a longer period of time; control rats developed tumors in 11 weeks, whereas fucoidan fed rats remained cancer free for 19 weeks.

In other studies, oral and intravenous doses of brown seaweed proved from 61% to 95% effective in preventing the development of cancer in rats implanted with sarcoma cells. One group of researchers described fucoidan as a "very potent anti-tumor agent in cancer therapy" after it inhibited the growth and spread of lung cancer in rats. (That type of cancer is particularly resistant to chemotherapy).

Various studies further demonstrated that fucoidan combats cancer in multiple ways:

>*It causes certain types of rapidly growing cancer cells (including stomach cancer, colon cancer and leukemia) to self-destruct (apoptosis).

*It physically interferes with cancer cell's ability to adhere to tissue. Thus it prevents the cancer from spreading (metastasizing) to other areas.

*It enhances production of microphages (white blood cells that destroy tumor cells), gamma interferon (proteins that activate microphages and natural killer cells), and interleukin (compounds that regulate the immune system).

PROOF FROM THE PANELISTS PRACTICE

But as Dr. Makise points out, fucoidan still needs to prove itself in large, double blind clinical trials involving creatures more evolved than guinea pigs. He believes there is compelling evidence that fucoidan can help prevent cancers. He has seen in Japan where fucoidan has helped patients with cancer already. He suggests cancer patients take combinations with it:

*AHCC or other immune enhancing mushrooms

*antioxidants, especially large doses of Selenium

*Enterococcus faecalis, beneficial bacteria found in the intestine— to control the bile acids and enhance vitamins as biotin and certain B vitamins.

*triple the amount daily of essential vitamins and minerals, and cancer patients take daily supplements of selenium and zinc.

*a healthy lifestyle and diet that avoids meat, milk and other animal proteins and fat. He recommends the synergistic effect of these foods.

2. A HEALING TREE FROM THE JUNGLES OF THE AMAZON: THE GRAVIOLA TREE (I personally take this product)

"Recently HSI uncovered a remarkable story about a natural cancer killer that has been kept under lock and key for over 20 years. There's a healing tree that grows deep within the Amazon rainforest in South America that could literally change how you, your doctor and probably the rest of the world think about curing cancer. It's called Graviola. Since the 1970s the bark, leaves, roots, fruit and fruit seeds of the Graviola Tree were studied in laboratory tests and with remarkable results."

Several years ago, a major pharmaceutical company began extensive independent research on it. They learned that certain extracts from the tree actually seek out, attack and destroy cancer cells. However since the natural extracts themselves could not be patented, the company labored to create a synthetic copy that showed the same results. After more than seven years of work behind closed doors, researchers at this company realized they couldn't duplicate the tree's natural properties with a patentable substance. So they shut down the entire project. It basically came down to this—if they couldn't make huge profits, they would keep the news of this possible cancer cure a well-guarded secret. But one researcher couldn't bear that, and decided to risk his job with the hope of saving lives.

SEVEN YEARS OF SILENCE BROKEN

This conscience-driven researcher contacted Raintree Nutrition, a natural products company dedicated to harvesting plants from the Amazon. In the course of working with Raintree on another story, they shared the exciting Graviola breakthrough with us. Since then, we've been looking closely on the research to date with Graviola. One of the first scientific references to it in the United States was by the National Cancer Institute (NCI). In 1976, the NCI showed that the stems and the leaves of this tree were effective in attacking and destroying malignant cells. But these results were part of the internal NCI report and were, for some reason, never made public.

Since 1976 there have been several promising cancer studies on Graviola. However, the tree's extracts have yet to be tested on cancer patients. No double-blind clinical trials exist, and clinical trials are typically the benchmark mainstream doctors and journals use to judge a treatment value. Nevertheless, our research has uncovered that Graviola has been shown to kill cancer cells in at least 20 laboratory tests.

The most recent study, conducted in Catholic University of South Korea, revealed that two chemicals extracted from Graviola seeds showed comparable results to the Chemotherapy drug Andramyacin when applied to malignant breast and colon cells in test tubes.

Another study, published in the Journal of Natural Products, showed Graviola is not only comparable to Andramyacin, but dramatically outperforms it in laboratory tests. Results showed it selectively killed colon cancer cells at "10,000 times the potency of Andramyacin."

Another ongoing treatment research is being supported by NCI (believe it or not) at Purdue University. The research is showing it is particularly effective against prostate and pancreatic cancer cells. In a separate study, Purdue researchers showed that extracts from the leaves of Graviola are extremely effective in isolating and killing lung cancer cells.

Perhaps the most significant result of the studies we have researched is that Graviola selectively seeks out and kills cancer cells—leaving all healthy, normal cells untouched. Chemotherapy (not therapy, they are poisons) indiscriminately seeks and destroys all actively reproducing cells, even normal hair and stomach cells, causing such devastating side effects as hair loss and severe nausea.

If you want more details on these studies, you can buy the Graviola Technical Report from either HIS, or from Saga Press direct. Grown and harvested by indigenous people in Brazil, Graviola is available on a limited supply in the United States, and is distributed through "Raintree Nutrition." It is suggested you consult with someone like Dr. Ward Joiner before using it, especially since, when combined with 7 other herbs, it would be much more effective. He also has the product in his warehouse for anyone to purchase. I also encourage you to consult with your regular M.D. before beginning any new therapy, especially when treating cancer.

I began using Graviola a year ago, combined with seven immune-boosting herbs, as a preventive along with all the other products and foods I consume. I am happy to say I have never suffered any side effects from the herbs I have taken by Dr. Joiner's recommendations.

3. HYBRIDIZED MUSHROOM EXTRACT DESTROYS CANCER CELLS AND PROVIDES POWERFUL IMMUNE PROTECTION

Until now, the only way to get access to this remarkable immune booster was to live in Japan. For the last five years in Japan, people with cancer, AIDS, and other life threatening diseases—as well as healthy people who want to stay that way—have been destroying tumor cells with a powerful extract called AHCC (activated Hexose correlate compound). Now AHCC is available to consumers in the United States.

"AHCC is an extract of a unique hybridization of several kinds of medicinal mushrooms known for their immune-enhancing capabilities. On their own, each mushroom has a long medical history in Japan, where their extracts are widely prescribed by physicians. But when combined into a single hybrid mushroom, the resulting active ingredient is so potent that dozens of rigorous scientific studies have now established AHCC as one of the world's safe and most powerful immune stimulations."

In vitro, animal and human studies confirm it works against and, in some cases, even prevents the recurrence of liver cancer, prostate cancer, ovarian cancer, multiple myeloma, breast cancer, and AIDs, with no dangerous side effects. In smaller doses, AHCC can also boost the immune function of healthy people, helping to protect their infections.

CALLING UP YOUR FIRST LINE OF DEFENSE

Without our immune system, our bodies would be overrun by bacteria, viruses, parasites, fungi, and other invaders; infections would rapidly spread, and cancer cells would proliferate. Like a highly responsive and well-coordinated army, our immune system is composed of a variety of specialized cells that identify, seek out, and destroy microbes, pathogens, and tumor cells.

The body's "front line defense" are the phagocytes and NK (natural killer) cells, which respond quickly to potential threats. NK cells grab on to the surface of substances or the outer membranes of cancer cells and inject a chemical hand grenade (called a granule) into the interior. Once inside, the granules explode and destroy the bacteria or cancer cell within five minutes. Undamaged, an NK cell moves on to the next victim. In its prime, a NK cell can take on two cancer cells at the same time, speeding up the process.

Recent research shows that as we age, our immune systems function less efficiently. In particular, the ability of our NK cells to respond quickly and efficiently declines with age and illness. Health can deteriorate rapidly when this occurs. When NK activity is low, diseases like AIDS, cancer, immune deficiency, liver disorders, and various diseases can occur. We must remember that measurements of NK activity correlates with one's chances of survival, and anything that helps increase NK cell activity may help people treat, recover from, and/or prevent these illnesses.

RESEARCH FINDS REMARKABLE IMMUNE SYSTEM BOOST IN MULTIPLE WAYS

Scientific studies of the extract AHCC, published in peer-reviewed journals such as International Journal of Immunology, Anti-Cancer Drugs, and Society of Natural Immunity, have established the health benefits and safety of AHCC more conclusively than nearly any other natural supplement. What is especially remarkable about AHCC is it consistently and effectively boosts immune system function. Specifically it does the following:

*Stimulates cytokine (IL-2, IL-12, TNE, and INF) production, which stimulates immune function

*Increases NK cell activity against diseased cells as much as 300%

*Increases the formation of explosive granules with the NK cells.

*Increases the number and the activity of lymphocytes, increasing the T cells up to 200%

*Increases Interferon levels, which inhibits the replication of viruses and stimulates NK cell activity

*Increases the formation of TNF, a group of proteins that destroy cancer cells

These dramatic effects were seen in a 1995 Clinical Trial reported in the International Journal of Immunotherapy, showing that 3 grams of AHCC per day significantly lowered the level of tumor markers found in patients with prostate cancer, ovarian cancer, multiple myeloma, and breast cancer. This study documented complete remissions in six of 11 patients, significant NK activity in 9 of 11 patients, and T and B-cell activity levels also rose significantly.

Up until recently, AHCC was only available in Japan; however, it is now available in the United States. You should discuss this with your physician or your Holistic doctor for correct dosages. The main goal is to raise your NK level which can be seen in your blood results.

4. THE LACTOFERRIN MIRACLE

"We're on the verge of a major medical breakthrough with lactoferrin. Because of this unique extract, much of what we now consider state-of-the-art medicine, such as radiation, antibiotics and chemo, may eventually be seen as bloodletting. If lactoferrin proves to be as powerful as it promises to be, many deadly diseases that haunt our thoughts today will no longer frighten us."

WHERE DOES LACTOFERRIN COME FROM AND HOW DOES IT WORK?

From the moment you were born, lactoferrin – non-binding protein found in breast milk (colostrom) – was your first shield against infection and disease and your primary source of immune-system chemicals. The primary task of your immune system is to survey your body—organ by organ, tissue by tissue, cell by cell—to make sure that only the cells that are supposed to be there are there. When a healthy immune system recognizes a foreign substance—a virus or cancerous cell—it immediately fights to eliminate it.

WHAT IS SO MYSTERIOUS ABOUT PREGNANCY?

Until recently, scientists had been baffled by the fact that woman's body doesn't normally reject the fetus, which naturally contains the foreign antigens of the father. But the puzzle is beginning to unravel: science has discovered that shortly after conception, a woman's system is down-regulated.

This is why her body does not reject the fetus as "foreign" matter (for this reason, pregnant women would not take lactoferrin). Immediately after delivery, however, her body produces colostrums, or the first milk, which restores the immune system and provides healthy immune chemicals to the infant. Lactoferrin is the primary immune-system chemical in first milk.

Studies have shown that this first milk is the only source the infant can get with significant immune substances. Synthetic formulas can't offer the same nutritional, immunological, or physiological value, despite efforts to produce formulas that mimic breast milk.

UNRAVELING THE HEALING MYSTERY OF LACTOFERRIN

Lactoferrin has at least two specific immune-boosting functions:

*It binds to iron in your blood, keeping it away from cancer cells, bacteria, viruses, and other pathogens that require iron to grow. The lactoferrin protein is able to sequester and release iron as needed, under controlled conditions. This property helps prevent harmful oxidative reactions, making lactoferrin a powerful antioxidant.

*It activates very specific strands of DNA that turn on the genes which launch your immune response. This is such a rare and surprising action that there is no other protein like it. It is in a class by itself.

*Lactoferrin also contains antibodies against a wide range of bacteria, fungal, and protozoa pathogens. In fact the protein backs budding cancer cells or bacteria into a corner, starves them and sends out a signal to your white blood cells that says: "It's over here, come and get it."

State-of-the-art-techniques in cellular and molecular biology have recently allowed us to isolate lactoferrin from the first food of life. The commercially available preparation is in a form in which the food has not been chemically altered.

Lactoferrin has been widely used to support recovery from malignancies of animals. Numerous studies on rats and patient case histories have documented the benefits of lactoferrin in helping to combat many other kinds of malignancies. In fact, many Holistic practitioners use it by combining it with other immune-enhancing natural tumor-fighting therapies. In one case, a leukemia patient (labeled the worst case the Mayo Clinic had seen in 20 years) had his condition reversed with lactoferrin. His white blood cell count rose, and his problem disappeared. This seemingly "hopeless" case was transformed into a remarkable recovery.

Other case histories indicate that the negative effects of conventional treatments like chemo and radiation are drastically reduced or eliminated with supplemental lactoferrin. It is noted you can use lactoferrin in higher doses with these more critical cases.

WHAT ELSE CAN YOU USE IT FOR?

Other clinical and case studies have shown:

*It contains an anti-inflammatory molecule—which means it can help if you suffer from the pain of inflammation.

*It plays a role in lessening ocular disturbance, which means it may help with vision problem.

*Acts as a potent antimicrobial agent against *Candida albicans*.

*Shows potent antiviral activity, useful in reducing your susceptibility to viruses, including Herpes and HIV.

If you are wondering how safe lactoferrin is, remember it is nontoxic and tolerable by nursing infants.

Lactoferrin can be very useful in treatment of cancer patients, without fear of side effects. Again, always consult a Holistic doctor before using because it is a natural substance so large pharmaceutical companies cannot patent it. Veteran Holistic treaters such as Dr. Ward Joiner can access which might be the best company to buy from.

5. The next new discovery: STOP CANCER WITH A KILLER GRAPEFRUIT

There's new research emerging on MCP exhibiting anti-cancer abilities and shedding some light on just how it achieves these effects. In certain types of cancer like prostate, breast, colon, and lung, it is showing good results in animal and human studies. MCP comes from pulp and rinds of citrus fruits, like oranges and grapefruits, that they have been modified to produce shorter sugar chains. Thus, they are more readily absorbed in the intestinal tract and into the blood stream to fight cancer cells.

These sugar chains, glycans, are fundamental to cell communication, and they bind to lectins. Without going into the heavy chemistry, the sugar chains in MCP seem to target one specific lectin called Galectin-3 that plays an important part in cancer development. Why? Because Galectin-3, in recent studies, have shown to be elevated in cancer tissues as compared to healthy ones. This linkage has been found in many cancers: thyroid cancer, gastric cancer, pituitary cancer, breast cancer, and colorectal cancer. Galectin-3 plays a role in a variety of biological functions related to cancer, including tumor cell adhesion, angiogenesis, apoptosis, and metastasis.

The main point here is that the Galectin-3 kills off immune system cells that are attempting to attack the cancer cells, and it also performs a protective barrier around the cancer cells, shielding them from the effects of anti-cancer drugs and treatments like chemo or radiation.

MCP CLOGS THE CANCER-GROWTH PIPELINE

So what does this have to do with grapefruit pulp? MCP's sugar molecules block the protein's ability to bind to carbohydrates on other cancer cells and on healthy tissues by binding to the galectin-3 carbohydrate receptor at the C-terminal end themselves. With their binding sites all clogged up, the cancer cells can't clump together and can't metastasize by adhering to other areas. It's a perfect example of the sugar chains anti-adhesive properties.

There have been several significant animal and laboratory studies demonstrating MCP's potential to stop or slow metastases and even kill cancer cells. In one study, mice were fed MCP in their drinking water and then injected with human breast cancer cells or human colon cancer cells. In all cases, MCP effectively inhibited tumor growth, spontaneous metastasis, and angiogenesis—the process by which cells develop new blood vessels.

In the breast cancer portion of the study, the tumor volume in mice treated with MPC was 1/3 of that of the untreated mice. And none of the MPC-treated mice developed lung metastases, while 66% of the untreated mice had tumors on their lungs at the end of the study.

EFFECTIVE CANCER THERAPY WITH NO SIDE EFFECTS

It's an impressive body of evidence. The results seen in these studies rival the effects of many cancer drugs. But what makes MCP even better is that it doesn't appear to have any dangerous side effects. Fewer than five percent have loose stools from taking MCP due to soluble fiber content. However this can be managed by reducing the dose and slowly working back up to the recommended level. But compared to the toxic side effects of conventional cancer treatments, these problems are very minor.

If you are fighting cancer, be sure to work with your Nutritional doctor and, if you ask for Citrus pectin, be sure he recommends MCP as this modified type is the type researchers used to come up with their results. Certainly this can be one of the many products in you arsenal to fight the cancer.

Again, it's important to use MCP (modified citrus pectin) – not just regular citrus pectin—to obtains these results; studies have shown that only MCP has the ability to inhibit cancer cell adhesion and impact Galectin-3 activity. In fact, nearly all of the research on MCP's effects has been conducted with the same formula.

If you are fighting cancer, talk to your doctor about adding MCP to your treatment plan. It may help your body respond better to the treatment you're receiving. Or it may just give your body the boost it needs to help fight the disease on its own.

6. THE CANCER MIRACLE CURE THAT CAN LEAVE HEALTHY CELLS HEALTHY

"Sometimes it seems like if only we can find a miracle cure for cancer which is safe and effective. And a miracle is just what Dr. Marc Hidvegi believed he found when he patented Avemar, a fermented wheat germ extract. Studies have shown that Avemar reduces cancer recurrence, cuts off the cancer's energy supply, speeds cancer cell death, and helps the immune system identify cells for attack."

Back in World War I, Dr. Albert Szent-Gyorgyi (a Nobel Prize recipient in 1937 for his discovery of Vitamin C) had seen the effects of mustard gas up close and personal and was determined to find a safer alternative for cancer treatment. His goal was to prevent the rapid reproduction that is characteristic of cancer cells. He theorized that supplemental quantities of naturally occurring compounds in wheat germ, called DMBQ, would help to chaperone cellular metabolism, allowing healthy cells to assume a normal course but prohibiting potentially cancerous ones from growing and spreading. His early experiments, published in the Proceedings of the National Academy of Sciences USA in the 1960s, showed effects of naturally occurring and synthetic DMBQ against cancer cell lines, confirming his theory.

But it was then that the science community shifted its focus to killing cancers outright at any cost. His approach, seen as negotiating with the enemy as opposed to destroying it outright, was cast to the side. It wasn't until the Fall of Communism in Hungary in 1989 –when scientists were allowed for the first time to pursue independent, personal interests—that Dr. Hidvegi picked up where Dr.Szent-Gyorgyi left off. But when Hidvegi's funding ran out, it seemed as if the research would once again be set aside. He had no money, had no prospects, and his wife insisted he give up research and find a paying job.

They were desperate. Yet he still had one thing at that time—faith. Being a devout man, he prayed to the Virgin Mary for guidance—and an investor. Miraculously, the very next day a stranger wrote Hidvegi a check somewhere in the $100,000 range. With that money he was able to patent a technique of fermenting wheat germ with baker's yeast. He named this fermented product Avemar in tribute to the Virgin Mary (Ave meaning hail and Mar meaning Mary). It became the standard compound for research and later commercialization, sincec it assured a longer shelf life while maintaining its live food status.

Avemar is supported by more than 100 reports (written for presentation or publication) conducted in the U.S., Hungary, Russia, Australia, Israel, and Italy and is validated by more than 20 peer-reviewed publications describing in vitro, in vivo, and human clinical trials.

Since 1996, over 100 studies done on Avemar have impressed Oncologists and cancer researchers. Studies have shown that when Avemar is used as an adjunct treatment, it enhances the effects of the standard treatment agents. It is particularly effective in reducing the chances of cancer recurrence.

In a controlled study, 170 subjects with primary colorectal cancer either had surgery and standard care with chemotherapy or the same plus 9 grams of Avemar taken once a day. Only 3 % of the people in the Avemar group experienced a recurrence, vs. more than 17 % of those in the chemo only group. The Avemar group also showed a 67% reduction in metastisis and a 62% reduction in death.

In a randomized study, 46 stage III Melanoma patients with a high risk of recurrence either had surgery and standard care with chemo, or surgery plus standard care and 9 grams of Avemar taken once a day. Those taking Avemar showed a 50% reduction in risk of progressive.

In a one year non-randomized trial of 43 patients with oral cancer, 21 patients received surgery and standard care while 22 others received the same plus Avemar. The Avemar group showed an 85% reduced risk of overall progression. Plus, only 4.5% of the patients in the Avemar group experienced local recurrences as opposed to more than 57 % of the people in the standard care group.

Avemar also reduced the frequency and severity of many common side effects, including nausea, fatigue, weight lost and immune suppression.

AVEMAR CUTS OFF CANCER CELL'S ENERGY SUPPLY

One of Avemar's most unique benefits is that it cuts off cancer cell's energy supply by selectively inhibiting glucose metabolism. Cancer cells love glucose – it fuels the voracious growth and spread of tumors. In fact, cancer cells utilize glucose at a 10 to 50 times higher rate than normal cells do.

Cancer cells that have a higher rate of glucose utilization have a greater chance of spreading. It's on these cells what we see Avemar's most dramatic effects. In fact, the greater the metastatic growth potential of the cancer cell line tested, the higher the glucose utilization rate and the more dramatic Avemar's effect.

Typical cancer treatments like chemo kill off cells—cancerous and healthy ones alike. But because of how Avemar interacts with glucose, it can selectively attack cancer cells while leaving healthy cells alone. Studies also revealed it would take a 50 times higher concentration of Avemar than is in a normal therapeutic dose to inhibit glucose utilization in normal healthy cells.

AVEMAR HASTENS CANCER CELL DEATH

The second way Avemar works against cancer is to keep cancer cells from repairing themselves. Cancer cells reproduce quickly and chaotically, producing many breaks in the cellular structure. Because of this, cancer cells need a lot of the enzyme known as PARP (poly-ADP-ribose) to repair breaks in DNA before the cells divide. Without adequate PARP, cancer cells cannot complete DNA replication. When there is no PARP to repair the damage, an enzyme called Caspace-3 initiates programmed cell death. Avemar has been known to speed up the death of cancer cells by inhibiting the production of PARP and enhancing the production of Caspace-3.

Researchers at UCLA also showed that Avemar reduces the production of RNA and DNA associated with the rapid production of cancer cells. It also restores normal pathways of cell metabolism and increases the production of RNA and DNA associated with healthy cells.

POSSIBLE GOOD NEWS FOR CHILDREN WITH CANCER USING AVEMAR

One of the most powerful studies on Avemar shows its effectiveness with children with cancer. One of the limiting factors in using chemo to treat children is the infection that can occur during treatment. Infections often set in because chemo kills large numbers of the child's infection-fighting white blood cells, and destroys many of the bone marrow cells that produce them.

Doctors aware of the immune-enhancing properties of Avemar wanted to learn if it could possibly prevent the life-threatening infections that often occur in pediatric patients. A recent study published in the medical journal Pediatric Hematology showed that such infections and the fever that accompanies them were reduced by 42 % in the children given Avemar after chemotherapy, compared to those not getting Avemar.

Avemar has this effect because it helps rebuild the immune system, increasing the number and activity of functioning of immune system cells.

It's clear that, unlike conventional cancer therapy, Avemar does not produce side effects – in fact, it reduces them.

Avemar will not hurt the rest of your body either. In fact, according to an independent panel of medical, food safety, and toxicology experts: "Avemar is as safe as whole wheat bread."

In Hungary, where it was developed and is manufactured, it is classified as a dietary food for special medical problems, and is a standard therapy for those with cancer. It is used as a dietary substance in other countries too.

It is important to note this product is a wheat product and no one should self feed themselves without consultation with an M.D. or Holistic doctor. People with other complications should always consult with a doctor before using Avemar. It is taken in the form of drink and, when used daily, a person could experience an effect within three weeks, reporting improvements in "appetite, energy, and general quality of life."

THIS CONCLUDES THE SIX BREAKTHROUGH SUPPLEMENTS. Aren't they truly amazing! It is hoped that someday soon medical doctors will follow more closely, and utilize, some of these amazing products.

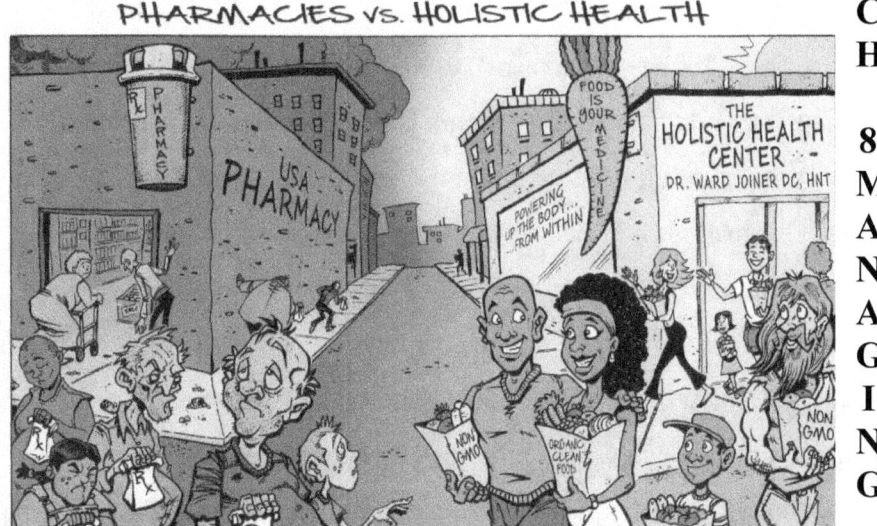

PHARMACIES VS. HOLISTIC HEALTH

NCER: LOOKING AT WHAT DOESN'T WORK

First, the FDA is a confusing entity. The Federal Drug Agency exists primarily to protect Americans against fraudulent, unethical and false claims of pharmaceutical companies, individuals who pretend/allege to have cures (when they don't), and are regulators of what is allowed or approved so that companies can market their chemical products. Historically they became a little involved in the research of Naturopathic doctors in the past, however overall they shun away from such involvement with herbs, plants and natural remedies for cancer prevention or cures. In a word, I see them as a two edged sword: helping on the one edge, harming by either allowing dangerous drugs on the market, or siding with pharm companies who have never proven their products—to the point of causing deaths or causing long term harm to the bodies of cancer patients.

One only has to watch some of the ludicrous and bizarre ads on TV today to realize the so-called remedies for many bodily dysfunctions are a bad joke. When they warn us of 10-20 potential side effects for a particular drug, and then a few years later it is pulled by them from the market, it makes all of us question the accuracy and the integrity of this agency. Avastin is a drug which had been approved by the FDA and subsequently prescribed by physicians for women with breast cancer. Recently the FDA banned it from use for said purpose. It was proven it did not reduce the progression of cancer and did not improve the health of women in any way. Just recently the FDA uncovered that doctors were prescribing it for their patients when the drug was imported from foreign manufacturers. A Federal warning was sent to Genentech Company to stop making it or be subject to criminal prosecution. And of course doctors were warned also.

This is but one of the countless violations by the FDA and pharms who place the cancer patients at risk daily, monthly and annually. It still perplexes me how they still are able to continue the assault on cancer victims with chemo drugs and radiation. My own doctor told me the other day that more acidity takes place in the body with radiation than with the drugs injected! We are talking about long term use of poisonous drugs in an attempt to target cancer cells. It is widely known this imposition on patients lowers the functions of the immune cells, the NK cells, T cells and IGF-1 proteins (which are intended to "energy up" the body in order to fight malignancies). It actually lessens the chances of a recovery since it is robbing the body of necessary nutrients. I have read the opinions of many doctors recently who have enough good research data to be able to predict that these pharm drugs will become a thing of the past shortly.

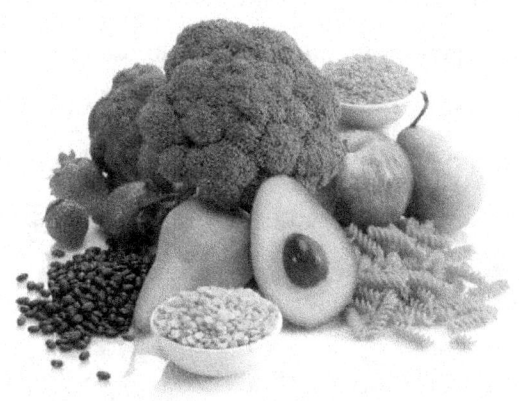

CH 9

HOW LACK OF FIBER CAN CAUSE MORE DISEASES

In spite of all the ads and articles on the dangers of lack of fibers in our bodies, Americans go on eating the same way they have always eaten. Our daily diets are chuck full of empty calories, refined foods, and loads of sugar and virtually very little of whole foods. When it comes to fiber, many of us make the mistake of believing that eating our daily bowl of Wheaties is a more than adequate source of fiber.

Sad to say, many of our pantries contain lots of white flour products, cooked and canned vegetables, cookies, chips and all those other brightly packaged foods that make you feel like you've reached that place of food utopia. These foods are usually fiber-less and have been artificially altered from their original state; many are more like "nonfoods."

Typical American eating habits have led to our lives being plagued with chronic constipation, intestinal gas, bowel disorders and a whole host of infections. And if one thinks that what goes on down there in our bowels is not related to our overall health, we are deluding ourselves. The truth is that our ability to expedite waste materials from the body is one of the great predictors of how healthy we are. And it is the fiber in our food choices which will determine how that predictor will have a negative or positive outcome.

WHAT EXACTLY IS FIBER?

Many of us have heard it is called "roughage" and is technically a food component that remains undigested as it passes through the gastrointestinal tract. It readily absorbs water and helps to add to the bulk required to form a good bowel movement. It is also described as a complex carbohydrate consisting of a polysaccharide and a lignin substance that gives structure to the cell of a plant. It is the portion of plant food which is not digested. Insoluble fiber has the ability to pass through the intestines intact and virtually unchanged. It has no caloric value and, unlike fats, carbohydrates and proteins, fiber does not provide the body with nutrients or fuel for energy. Dietary fiber is only found in plant components, such as vegetables, fruits and whole grains.

SOLUBLE FIBER is the fiber which will be digested in the large intestine, so its bulking power is limited. Soluble fibers can dissolve in water and provide many positive features:

**helps prevent blood sugar highs and lows

**helps lower blood cholesterol

**lowers the risk of heart disease

**helps to control high blood pressure

**encourages friendly bacteria to grow

INSOLUBLE FIBER possesses these positive benefits:

**keeps the bowel clean and operative

**helps bind dangerous toxins and hormones for better excretion

**fosters regularity

**help us to digest our food better

**prevents constipation

**helps lower the risk of bowel disease

SOURCES OF SOLUBLE FIBER are found in pectin, lignin, gums and mucilages, bean, apples, pears, oat bran. It is digestible and when broken down it creates a kind of gel as it absorbs water in the intestinal tract. Unlike the soluble fiber, it does not bulk the stool, and it does have a tendency to slow down the rate it is digested. Soluble fibers are also found in vegetables such as onions, bulbs, leeks, and asparagus. Fruits, including dried fruits, are soluble fibers.

SOURCES OF INSOLUBLE FIBER are primarily composed of cellulose, a non-digestible form of fiber found in the outer portions of vegetables and fruits. In addition, the bran or seed covering of whole grains is another source of insoluble fiber. Hemicellulose fibers have the ability to remain unchanged and absorb water as they travel in the digestive tract. They increase stool bulk and transit time and prevent constipation and conditions like hemorrhoids. Interestingly enough, the insoluble fiber content of fruits is found in its flesh and stringy membranes rather than the peelings.

I didn't realize these statistics on fibers until I got cancer and began studying healthy foods:

We need at least 35 grams daily of fiber. The average American consumes 9 grams of fiber daily. If we want to live a long and healthy life, those stats have got to change. The reason is because fiber has these benefits:

**Increase fecal bulk by retaining water

**Decreases stool transit time

**keeps blood sugar levels more stable

**Helps prevent weight gain by slowing the rate of digestion and helps control hunger

**Expedites the removal of toxins and carcinogens from the bowels

**binds with bile salts, which can help with the risk of gall bladder disease and certain types of cancer

**Creates the presence of healthier intestinal bacteria

Until I got my cancer I did not realize what diseases are being caused by the lack of fibers in our diets. Recent stats from dietary experts are emphasizing the linkage of low fiber to appendicitis, attacks, inability of the body to get rid of excess estrogens (or upsetting the hormonal balance), heart disease, and high cholesterol levels.

CH 10
FOODS TO EAT, FOODS TO AVOID AND BODY pH
FACTOR ACID-ALKALINE BALANCE

Why is it important to focus on foods which create an acidic state in the body as opposed to an alkaline state? Very simply, it could be a matter of life and death. There is a preponderance of evidence in medicine today that cancers love to feed off acidity in the body, and will die in an alkaline state. It was not in my awareness of the existence of these two conditions until after my surgery and I began doing my research. My blood tests were showing a reading of 4.5 (highly acidic); so I wanted to learn how to improve it.

I began by exploring the internet, talking to Alden at the Sunrise Natural Food Store in Roseville, CA, learned I needed to buy some litmus paper so that I could test my own saliva at home (you can also test your urine). I even tested city water in Sacramento and Roseville, discovering both were acidic at 6.0. At a supermarket I discovered Fiji Water from the islands of Fiji; each bottle shows 7.5 alkaline. It is water that has passed through volcanic ash for ages and thus it retains this perfect alkaline state. After that I learned about the Kangen machine, one of many reverse osmosis machines which can produce up to a 9.0 reading.

In this chapter I have listed the foods which help us maintain an alkaline balance suitable for good health, and another list of acid producing foods which are detrimental to those of us with a cancer diagnosis.

THE FOLLOWING IS ONLY A PARTIAL LIST. I CONSUME MOST OF THESE FOODS ON THE ALKALINE SIDE AND AVOID THE OTHERS.

ALKALINE-PRODUCING

Watermelons

Lemons

Orange juice

Broccoli

Raspberries

Spinach

Blueberries

Dandelion seeds

Veggies (dark greens)

Strawberries

Pineapples

Mg, Fe, K

Celery

Artichokes

Bok Choy

Lettuce

Onions

Walnuts

Pecans

Shitake mushrooms

Egg plant

Organic fresh herbs

Avocados

Turkey, chicken

Sunflower seeds

Organically farmed fish

White bass

Pacific cod

Cold water Prawns

Tilapia

Stevia (a natural sweetener)

BEVERAGES

Lemon in water

All Natural herbal teas

Sugar free syrups for waffles and pancakes

Mild Coffee (not heavily caffeinated)

ACID-PRODUCING FOODS

Red meats

Beans

Prunes

Most grains

Cranberries

Plums

Eggs

Gravy

Distilled water

Aged cheeses

Hot dogs

Pastrami

Sausages

Ham

Butter, Cream, Ice cream

Sour cream

Super-heated vegetable oils

Barbeque sauces

Mustard

Caffeine

Baker's yeast

Brewers' yeast

SWEETENERS

Artificial sweeteners

Barley

Brown sugars, corn syrup, glucose

Granulated sugar

Most colas, i.e. Pepsi, Coca colas, Squirt, etc.

(Due to high sugar contents)

Again, this is a partial list of foods to consider. They worked for me on the whole. Also, I suggest you consult the data of the Price Pottinger Foundation.

In conclusion, if a food causes acidity in the system, it is labeled an acid-producing food. If it increases the pH to 7.0+, it is an alkaline-producing food. The effect some foods have on urine pH may be quite different than the food itself; for example, lemon is considered highly acidic by itself, but after eaten, it becomes alkaline (as the body metabolizes it to cause the blood to become alkalized). If one has cancer it is important to know these things so you can learn how to be in control of the pH factors. This can be also true for other diseases, so be sure to consult with your Nutritionist or Naturopath. In general, the medical doctors won't tell you to stay away from certain foods. Instead, they pretend their Allopathic formula for cancer will work. Not so. This is why I won't accept their perception of Naturopathic ways. They appear to want to remain ignorant. They don't want to think outside the box of their own thinking. When they wake up it is usually when they, or a close relative, is diagnosed with cancer.

For even more insight and understanding I suggest you read: THE ACID-ALKALINE FOOD GUIDE, a quick reference to foods and their effects on pH levels, by Dr. Susan E. Brown, PhD, CCN, and a New York certified Nutritionist and Researcher. Her co-author is Larry Trivieri, an author who co-authored a book Alternative Medicine: The Definitive Guide – probably the most complete guide to which foods make your system acid-producing and which will help you achieve an alkaline state.

The essence of his book is aptly stated, to which I adhere: Both health and disease begin in the cells, for it is at the cellular level that the vast majority of the body's multitude of interactions occur.

For example, in order for the body's cells to function properly, they need to receive life giving nutrients and oxygen from the bloodstream and, at the same time, they need to release cellular wastes. Only when the body is in an alkalized state can it assimilate good nutrients and expel wastes. When the body becomes chronically acidic, however, these and many other cellular processes start to become impaired. Eventually if acidity remains unchecked, the combination of a diminished oxygen supply to the cells, and a buildup of wastes inside the cells sets into motion both fatigue and disease.

In summary, this was perhaps the most significant discovery since my cancer diagnosis: THAT CONTROLLING THE ALKALINE STATE IN OUR BODIES IS THE MAIN KEY TOWARD ENABLING THE HEALTHY CELLS TO KILL THE LITTLE ENEMIES. As my Holistic Doc Joiner told me when we first met: "I am not in the business of curing cancers. What seems to be the case is that a healthy immune system is like the old Pac Man game when computers were invented: it is just knocking out cancers one at a time." He always added: "in the final analysis it is the body which heals itself, no single situation, chemical, or circumstance in itself." As he repeated: "we don't cure cancers, we help folks rebuild their healthy cells, strengthen them, maintain them – so the body can heal itself."

CH 11
NANO SILVER SOL FOR YOUR CANCER AND OTHER DISEASES

This liquid is a new broad spectrum, anti-bacterial, antiviral and anti-fungal solution. I am mentioning it here because I have had personal success with it. This new antimicrobial was patented in 2006, is backed by a growing body of scientific study, and is increasingly used in clinical applications.

This Silver Sol is quickly becoming a popular alternative to synthetic antibiotics. I had a weakened immune system the second year after my cancer surgery and I picked up an infection on my knee at a Fitness Center where I was working out. My knee swelled to 3 times its size so I immediately visited my dermatologist. When he saw it his face showed a look of fright and he said I must immediately report to the hospital emergency room for diagnosis and recommended treatment. The doctor there drained it to reduce the swelling. The lab diagnosis indicated it was MRSA, one of the worst hospital infections known, and indicated many folks die from it and/or require days of hospitalization with heavy antibiotics.

Having studied about Nano Silver sol and being confident it could heal my infection, I returned to the dermatologist's office for a discussion. He wanted to prescribe an antibiotic. I told him that I no longer care to use antibiotics because it is not the best solution, since I was a cancer patient at the time. I explained to him that Silver sol solution was my natural treatment of choice. He became very angry at me and said: "I have studied the material for years about MRSA and antibiotics are all that is effective." He stormed out of the room because he felt I wasn't adhering to his choice of treatment, and returned ten minutes later after he gained his composure!

The good news: the Nano silver sol solution was effective. Within 3-5 days the swelling shrunk and ten days later it healed completely. My wife had mixed feelings about my choice; however I had done the research and was convinced on how best to treat the problem. This is just one example of how my choices have made the difference in my overall health issues.

Even though I used Guardian company Silver sol initially, there are other companies that now market it. One of my favorite sites on the internet is the video of Dr. Gordon Pederson of Guardian silver sol.com, wherein he explains the uses of the product, including that it may kill cancers.

Though there are about 90 different uses for this amazing product, here is a short list of possible cures:

Abcesses, athletes foot, acne, antibacterial, antifungal (and some doctors believe cancer is a fungus), antitumor, antiviral, antibiotic alternative, bladder infection, boils, bronchitis, burns, canker sores (it cured mine too), cavities, colds, colitis, diarrhea and dysentery, Epstein-barr virus, genital herpes(this worked effectively on a lady friend of mine), Immune modulator, IBS Irritable Bowel Syndrome, Leprosy, liver disease, Malaria (children in Africa are now being treated and cured!), Lupus, Prostate disease, rashes, rosacea, sore throat, Tuberculosis, vaginal odor, warts and yeast.

It can be consumed by drinking, tastes like water, or topically in many cases.

A few words about "antifungal": Fungus can get into any warm, moist area and often feeds off sugars. Cutting off sugars can combat intestinal fungus or yeast. For such infections in the armpits or vagina, apply silver sol directly to the yeast or take it internally.

Yeast and fungus can get into your intestines, causing muscle pain and symptoms of depression and attention deficit disorder. It can also result in all the symptoms of headaches, lymph problems, lupus and autoimmune disorders, including fibromyalgia. Silver sol has been used as colonic in the rectum, and douches are being successful in the vagina.

What about Nano silver sol as an antitumor? Tumors can have a myriad of causes. One bacterium is not usually the cause of a tumor, but when bacteria get into the cells and neutralize your immune function, you become more susceptible to other toxins in the air and water. This allows the DNA to be damaged and a tumor to form. Bacteria such as Hepatitis B can cause cancer. Viruses can also cause tumors and cancer, including the human papilloma virus that can result in cervical cancer in women.

This is one of the "miracle" discoveries I came across since diagnosed with cancer. It is unbelievable in a way! It is the only known cure for malaria which runs rampant and kills millions in Africa to this day. The medical profession in the U.S. doesn't prescribe it because it is a natural product—so talking to most of them about it is just about a waste of effort and time. They only want to hear about "cures" if it is chemically made in laboratories and then sold at a high price.

Again, as in important reminder, always make sure you are consulting with a Holistic or Naturopathic doctor when using this product. If you are under the care of an M.D. simultaneously, it is best to keep him abreast of your knowledge and intentions with Nano Silver Sol.

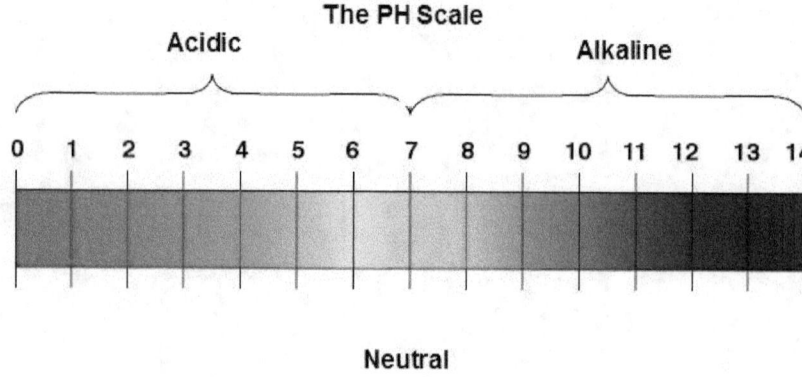

The PH Scale

Acidic

Alkaline

0 1 2 3 4 5 6 7 8 9 10 11 12 13 14

Neutral

CH 12

ASSESSING MY OWN pH AS A STEP TO BETTER HEALTH

Water is the most abundant compound in the human body, comprising 70% of the body. The body has an alkaline-acid ratio called the pH which is a balance between positively charged ions (acid forming) and negatively charged ions (alkaline forming). The body continues to strive to balance pH. When the balance is upset, many problems can occur.

How can one test his pH? By using pH test strips which you can buy at any natural food store. It is recommended you test your pH levels to determine if your body's pH needs immediate attention. I began testing myself early on after my cancer diagnosis. It was very low at 5.5. When the body tests 6.8-7.3, it is within normal range. It is best to test yourself one hour before a meal and two hours after a meal. In my case it took 6 months to restore a corrected saliva balance.

URINE pH

The results of urine testing indicate how well your body is assimilating minerals, especially calcium, magnesium, sodium and potassium. These are called the "acid buffers" because they are used by our body to control the acid level. If the acid level is too high the body will not be able to excrete acid. It must either store the body in tissues (auto-toxication) or buffer it – that is, borrow mineral from organs, bones, etc. in order to neutralize acidity.

SALIVA pH

You will also want to test the pH of your saliva. The results of saliva testing indicate the activity of digestive systems in your body, especially in the liver and stomach. This reveals the flow of enzymes running through your system shows the effects on all body systems.

WHAT CAUSES ME TO BE ACIDIC?

The reason acidosis is so common in our society is mostly due to the typical American diet, which is far too high in acid-producing animal products like meat, eggs, and dairy, and far too low in alkaline-producing foods like fresh vegetables. We also tend to eat acid-producing processed foods such as white flour and sugar products, as well as beverages like coffee and high sugar soft drinks. We use too many drugs which are acid-producing, and we use artificial chemical sweeteners like Nutrasweet Equal, and Aspartame. It is becoming rather enlightening to realize correcting an over acidic body by cleaning up our lifestyle can save us from many possible diseases. By the way, I use Stevia as my sweetener, a natural, harmless, tasty substitute.

In my case I was eating too many donuts, candies, milk shakes, pies, and just about 90% of what I ate had huge amounts of sugar in it. I was an acid monster, in retrospect a full blown sugar addict. On my red blood cell test, the cells were scoring a five on a one to five scale, one being eating low amounts of sugar. On top of that I wasn't hydrating enough (drinking sufficient water), not to forget the fact I did not know at the time water from the tap is acidic. Later on I learned the importance of drinking alkalized water (which I consume everyday now). Remember science has now well documented that cancer love to eat acids, and die in an oxygen state. I quit eating red meats, less cheese and less milk products, and less carbs. I prefer the dark green veggies because they are antioxidants and are easy to digest. We cancer patients must alkalize, alkalize, alkalize!! I suggest you don't over alkalize though.

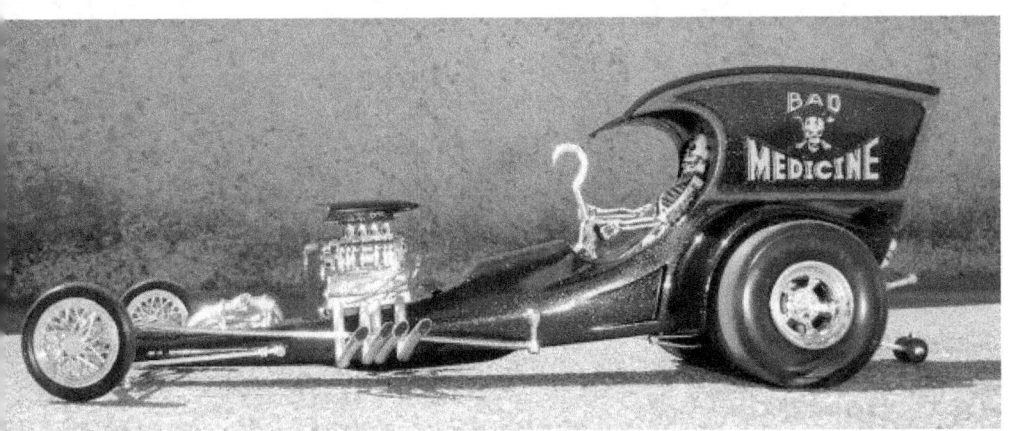

CH 13
WHY MEDICINE WON'T ALLOW CANCER TO BE CURED

We are reminded by Dr. Mercola in a fascinating documentary how terribly destructive is the epidemic of cancer in America today. He states in Mercola.com: "Imagine a commercial plane crashed and there were some fatalities involved. You can be sure that would make the headline of every major newspaper. Well, we have the equivalent of 8-10 planes crashing EVERY DAY with everyone on board dying from cancer. Nearly two million Americans are diagnosed with cancer every year – one person out of three will be hit with a cancer diagnosis at some time in their lives, in spite of the massive technological advances over the past half a century. Western medicine is no closer to finding a "cancer cure," while cancer has grown into a worldwide epidemic of staggering proportions. The statistics speak for themselves:

* In the early 1900s, one in twenty people developed cancer

* In the 1940s, one in 16 people

* In the 1970s, one in 10.

*Today, it's one in 3!

According to the FDC, about 1,660,290 new cancer cases are expected to be diagnosed in 2014. If overall death rates are falling, why are incident rates still on the rise? The answer is simple: the 40 year "war on cancer" has been a farce.

The cancer epidemic is a dream for Big Pharmas, and their campaign to silence cancer cures have been fierce, which is a tale well told in the documentary film: "Cancer, Forbidden Cures."

Indeed cancer is a big business. The cancer industry's focus is on earning billions, not dealing in effective prevention strategies, such as dietary guidelines, obesity, education and exercise. Instead it pours money into treating cancer, not preventing or curing it. Again, Mercola reminds us: "If the Pharmas can keep the well-oiled "cash cow" running they will continue to make massive profits on chemotherapy drugs, radiotherapy, diagnostic procedures and surgeries."

An average cancer patient spends $60,000 fighting the disease. Chemo drugs are among the most expensive of all treatments, ranging from $3,000 to $7,000 per month. If the cancer industry allows a cure with complimentary or alternative strategies, then their patient base goes away. For them it makes more sense to keep a steady stream of cancer patients alive but sick, and coming back for more.

Over the past hundred years, a number of natural cancer treatments have been developed and are used successfully to treat patients in the U.S. and other countries. All of them have been vehemently discounted by some doctors and pharmas, silenced and pushed under the rug. Physicians and researchers have been smeared, attacked and sent to prison for daring to defy the medical establishment.

Cancer patients deserve more. They deserve to be informed of the best alternative plants, vegetables, antioxidants, enzymes, amino acids, and of quality supplements. To limit them to only chemo poisons and radiation destruction of healthy cells is tragic, yet for some strange reasoning the conventional system dominates the scene.

Dr. Ward L. Joiner DC, HNT and Brandy Gillmore HNT
Holistic Nutritionists

Granite Bay Holistic Health Center

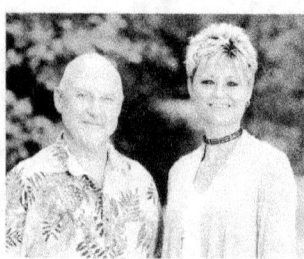

Dr. Ward Joiner DC, HNT and associate **Brandy Gillmore, HNT** are *Holistic Nutritionists* working at the cellular level to identify hormonal imbalances and immune deficiencies through blood lab testing and Live Blood Morphology. They offer their own unique holistic alternative protocols found nowhere else in the world. They specialize in strengthening immune systems and naturally balancing hormones including Testosterone, HGH and IGF-1 levels, so the body can naturally restore its own physiological balance. *Patients say they feel biologically younger and stronger, with an improved optimistic attitude, renewed mental clarity and recharged sexual desire/performance.*

Dr. Joiner's life health history represents a wide and varied spectrum of health challenges from a very young age. His proven and inspiring *modern holistic philosophy for renewed health* was developed with his insight of 30 years experience, education, personal research and clinical trials. He shares his simple, unique and proven protocols with patients worldwide, including those undergoing or recovering from life-threatening illnesses to those ecstatic about reversing the symptoms of aging or simply optimizing their health. Dr. Joiner has proven his protocols in immune science and anti-aging (in some cases reverse-aging), considered by some mainstream medical practitioners to be a modern miracle.

Dr. Joiner's proprietary individual protocols start at a cellular level, naturally **Powering Up the Body**, providing a healthy pH, strengthening the immune system, balancing hormones and **Optimizing the Body's Elimination Systems** providing an effective body detoxification. His protocols "naturally" raise low testosterone (Low T), HGH and IGF-1 hormone levels for women and men of all ages. He utilizes *quantifiable blood lab results* from his patient's local blood labs to monitor their improved results.

Brandy Gillmore began studying holistic health more than eight years ago when she was faced with her own health crisis. Since overcoming this life-changing experience, she speaks internationally educating others on the critical importance of being aware and proactive in our own health choices. She utilizes an educational process, referred to as *Live Blood Morphology*, which allows people to view a sample of their own live blood to see imbalances or deficiencies in their body (see right). Based on the various abnormalities detected in the blood, she makes recommendations including dietary changes and beneficial supplementation to *optimize overall digestion, strengthen the immune system, and remove stressful imbalances from the body*. She works to restore balance and optimize the body's ability to heal itself, in addition to increasing vitality, mental clarity and an overall sense of well-being.

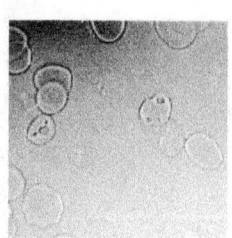

Celebrities, professional athletes, men, women and children of all ages comprise Gillmore's client-base. Her training includes Live Blood Morphology, Holistic Health, Nutritional Therapy, Neuro-linguistic Programming, Personal Training and Sports Nutrition. Her success in this field comes from an extraordinary protocol based from years of research, clinical trials and a completely unique perspective on the body and its inter-workings.

Granite Bay Holistic Health Center
8207 Sierra College Blvd., Suite 520 B
Granite Bay, CA 95661

www.MyHolisticHealth.net
Office 916.791.5555
Fax 916.791.5556

Dr. Ward L. Joiner DC, HNT and Brandy Gillmore HNT
Holistic Nutritionists

Dr. Joiner and associate **Brandy Gillmore** offer proprietary individual protocols starting at a cellular level, *Naturally Powering Up the Body*, providing a healthy pH, strengthening the immune system, balancing hormones and *Optimizing the Body's Elimination Systems* providing body detoxification. His protocols *naturally* raise low testosterone (Low T), HGH and IGF-1 hormone levels for women and men of all ages. He utilizes quantifiable blood lab results from his patient's local blood labs to monitor their improved results.

Naturally increasing Testosterone stimulates the body's own Human Growth Hormone (HGH) level, which activates the body's production of Insulin-like Growth Factor 1 (IGF-1) to optimal levels. Clinical studies prove this natural process facilitates repair and regeneration of damaged cells, strengthens the immune system, balances hormones, and slows or "reverses" aging. *Naturally* increasing Testosterone, HGH and IGF-1 levels is considered by some mainstream medical practitioners to be a modern miracle. Dr. Joiner's clinical studies continue to mystify medical society and further support his previous research. Many of Dr. Joiner's patients have had the following positive results and more, using his *all-natural* protocols.

- Increase Energy Stamina
- Achieve Better and Sounder Sleep
- Improve Your Optimistic Attitude & Mental Processes
- Strengthen the Immune System & Better Digestion
- Lower Blood Pressure and Cholesterol
- Regain Youthful Exuberance and Improved Outlook
- Increase Muscle Tone and Elasticity of the Skin
- Improved Cartilage Formation of the Joints
- Recharge Sexual Desire and Performance
- Regrow hair (in some cases) or reduce the gray
- Increase Muscle Mass and Loss Fat Content
- Increase Bone Mass / Reverse the Process Leading to Osteoporosis
- Speed Healing to Old Injuries and Improved Joint Mobility
- Diminish or Eliminate Cellulite and Wrinkles
- Promote Regeneration of Aged and Weakened Organs

Testosterone - The Master Hormone, by Dr. Ward L. Joiner D.C. clinical studies concludes Testosterone, HGH and IGF-1 hormone levels must be optimized *naturally* for these clinical results.

Doctors' Secrets The Road to Longevity, by Donald M. McCloud M.D. and Philip A. White M.D.,

Naturally Raising Your HGH Levels, by Dr. Dicken Weatherby N.D.

Granite Bay Holistic Health Center   www.MyHolisticHealth.net
8207 Sierra College Blvd.Suite 520 B   Office 916.791-5555
Granite Bay, CA 95661   Fax 916.791-5556

CH 14

THE TRUTH IS IN OUR BLOOD

I am showing you the brochure (front and back) of the Holistic Health Center in Roseville, CA, since these are the two top pros who were my coaches/guides to recovery over the past 5 years. Their mutual goal, which became mine, is to balance the immune system, the hormones including testosterone, HGH, and HGF-1 proteins so that my body could fight off and destroy the cancer pathogens invading my body.

Brandi specializes in doing red blood cell Morphology, which means she takes a prick of blood from the finger, places it under a high powered microscope, so that the patient can see his own live red blood cells analyzed on a TV monitor. She can then educate the person to any imbalances or deficiencies, then recommend certain foods or supplements to correct the problem. She works to restore balance and optimize the body's ability to heal itself. The cost of this procedure is very small when compared to the expensive machine processes used by the medical clinics or hospitals.

In my own case, over many months we saw blood cells which were distorted. Some examples include: lack of Vitamin B12, lack of water in my system, poor digestion of fats, the inability of my liver and kidney to fully assimilate foods. Note: every cancer patient has a damaged liver.

Then Dr. Joiner recommended supplements or educated me as to how to improve my food diet.

In summary, the truth of what was detrimental to my health was in this analysis of my own red blood cells. Doing it helped me relax, because once I saw the distorted picture on screen, it motivated me to take action to take the recommended correction from Ms. Gilmore and Dr. Joiner.

I strongly recommend this test for anyone who has any illness. It is simple, easy to do, practical and fast to implement for good results. It truly hastened my recovery from cancer.

Dr. Ward Joiner, DC, HNT & Brandy Gillmore, HNT
www.MyHolisticHealth.net
916.791.5555 / 877.948.5234

LIVE CELL NUTRITIONAL BLOOD ANALYSIS

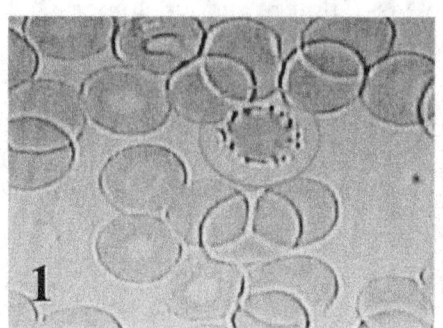

- Acanthocyte

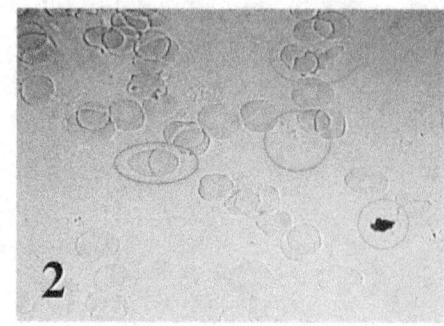

- Acanthocyte • Poikilocytosis
- Ovalcytes • Fungal Forms • Plaque

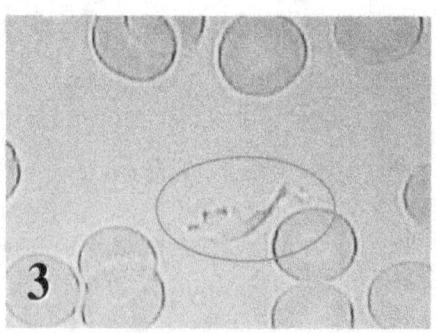

- Parasitized Red Blood Cell

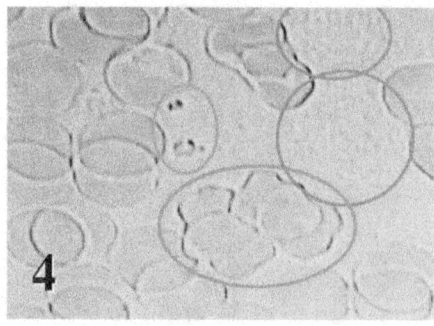

- Parasitized Red Blood Cell • White Blood Cells
- Poikilocytosis

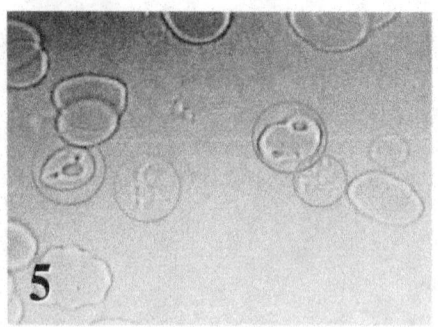

- Bacteria Infested Red Blood Cell
- Fungal Forms

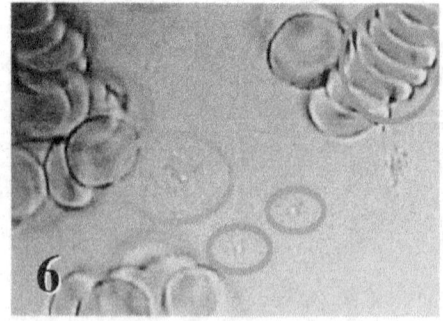

- Rouleau
- Fungal Forms • Sugar Crystals

CH 15
IF I HAVE CANCER, HOW MUCH SUGAR IS GOOD, HOW MUCH IS BAD?

We read frequently people saying "cancers love sugar" and are the biggest promoter of cancers. However, as we all know, fruits have sugar and have good vitamins and some even recommend we eat five kinds of fruit a day. These make nice intellectual discussions, but for the person with cancer it is somewhat scary and is certainly uncertain. So what to do?

SUGAR AS A TOXIC certainly needs examination and is there such a thing as good sugar? On May 26, 2009, Robert Lustig gave a lecture titled "Sugar: The Bitter Truth," which was posted on YouTube the following July. Since then, it has been viewed 800,000 times, a 90 minute discussion of the nuances of fructose biochemistry and human physiology.

Lustig is a specialist on pediatric hormone disorders and the leading expert on childhood obesity at the University of California, San Francisco School of Medicine, which is one of the best medical schools in the country. He published his first paper on childhood obesity a dozen years ago, and he has been treating patients and doing research on the disorder ever since.

The viral success of his lecture, according to Gary Taubes, an independent investigator in health policy with the Robert Wood Johnson Foundation independent, an affiliate with the New York Times Magazine group, has little to do with Lustig's impressive credentials and more to do with the persuasive case he makes that sugar is a "toxin" or a "poison", in addition to five references to sugar as merely "evil." Lustig means not only the white granulated stuff that we put in coffee or on cereal—technically known as sucrose—but also high-fructose corn syrup. "It's not about the calories," according to Lustig. "It's a poison in itself."

If Lustig is right, then our excessive consumption of sugar is the primary reason that the numbers of obese and diabetic Americans have skyrocketed in the past 30 years. It would also mean that sugar is also the cause of heart disease, hypertension, and many types of cancer. In his view, sugar should be thought of, like cigarettes and alcohol, as something that is killing us.

Taubes is not an M.D. nor a researcher, but he feels, based on years of researching and talking to many medical researchers and the data derived from them, that his conclusion is the same as Lustig's. But the big argument by opponents of this thinking is over what really is sugar.

What Lustig means by sugar is both sucrose—beet and cane sugar whether it is white or brown—and high fructose corn syrup—a processed food. In the early 1980s, corn syrup replaced sugar in sodas and other products because refined sugar then had the reputation as a noxious substance. Today high-fructose corn syrup is being portrayed by the food industry as a healthful alternative, and that's how the public perceives it. It was also cheaper than sugar. Now the tide is beginning to turn, and advertisements are promoting refined sugar by offering sucrose as the good food and advertising it by saying "No high-fructose corn syrup" in our products. Lustig of course is teaching both are poisonous and bad for our health.

Of course the argument from companies who produce sweetened beverages is that the real problem is people are consuming too much of it and getting sick.

There is only one study being done in this country, by Havel and Stanhope at the University of California at Davis, directly addressing the question of how much sugar is enough to trigger the symptoms of insulin resistance and metabolic syndrome. They are having healthy people drink 3 sugar or high-fructose beverages a day and then see the results. They sense that even over a short two week span they will see a reaction and symptoms of a metabolic syndrome.

CANCER AND METABOLIC SYNDROME (cancer causation)

The connection between obesity, diabetes, and cancer was first reported in large population studies by researchers from the WHO (World Health Organization) International agency for cancer for Research on Cancer. But since then, there is a plethora of theories and ideas about the relationship between insulin resistance, diabetes, fat in the liver, and the phenomenon medical professionals now label metabolic syndrome.

Let's talk about metabolic syndrome for a minute: the first symptom doctors are told to look for in diagnosing the syndrome is an expanding waistline. This means that if you are overweight, there is a good chance you have metabolic syndrome, and this is why you are more likely to have a heart attack or diabetes, or both, than someone who is not.

Having metabolic syndrome is another way of saying that the cells in your body are actively ignoring the action of the hormone insulin—a condition known technically as being insulin-resistant. And the reason this action of metabolic syndrome and insulin resistant get hardly any mention in the press, is cholesterol seems to get first attention.

Here is the explanation for this:

You secrete insulin in response to the food you eat—particularly the carbohydrates—to keep blood sugar in control after a meal. When your cells are resistant to insulin your body, your pancreas responds to rising blood sugar by pumping out more and more insulin. Eventually the pancreas can no longer keep up with demand and becomes exhausted. Now your blood will rise out of control, and you've got diabetes.

Having chronically elevated insulin levels has harmful effects of its own—heart disease. It results in higher triglyceride levels and high blood pressure, lower levels of HDL cholesterol (the good kind), and further worsening the insulin resistance: this is metabolic syndrome.

So the answer to the question as to whether sugar is as bad as Lustig says is it could very well be. It may be true that sugar and high fructose corn syrup, because of the way we metabolize fructose and at the levels we now consume it, cause fat to accumulate in our livers, followed by insulin resistance and metabolic syndrome. This then triggers the process that leads to heart disease, diabetes and obesity. They could indeed be toxic, but they take years to do their damage in most cases. We still need long term studies to know for sure how long it takes.

Now what is the connection for cancer to this process described above? This connection between obesity, diabetes and cancer was first reported in 2004 in large population studies by researchers from the WHO International Organization for Research on Cancer. It is not controversial. What it means is that you are more likely to get cancer if you are obese or diabetic than if you're not, and you are more likely to get cancer if you have metabolic syndrome. Of course all this ties to a study of the Western diet and life styles also.

It has been concluded by top researchers recently that insulin-growth factor creates tumors and promotes their growth. Craig Thompson, a top researcher at the Memorial Sloan-Kettering Cancer Center in New York, believes that many pre-cancerous cells would never acquire the mutations that turn them into malignant tumors if they weren't being driven by insulin to take up more blood sugar and metabolize it. This is particularly true in breast and colon cancers.

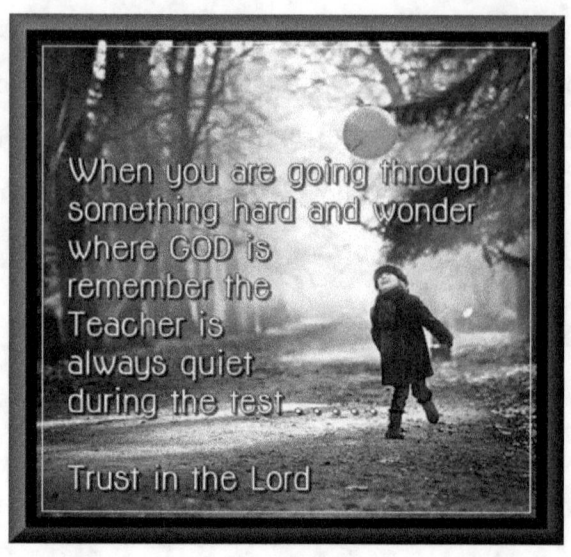

When you are going through something hard and wonder where GOD is remember the Teacher is always quiet during the test . . . .

Trust in the Lord

CH 16

OVERCOMING 10 VITAMIN DEFICIENCIES
COULD SAVE YOUR LIFE

There is nothing worse than to have a disease or deficiency and not to know the cause of the body's reaction. Basically the body needs all the essential vitamins, too much or too little can cause sickness. I will list just ten vitamins, the deficiency, the symptoms, and the name of the disorder, if it is serious.

Many of these are non-issues if you have a variety of foods you are eating, however it is important to know we must not lose focus on those vitamins we consume on a regular basis:

1. Vitamin A deficiency – night blindness or inability to see in dark places. It is found mainly in liver and carrots. Not common if you are eating a rounded diet.

2. Vitamin B5 deficiency – can cause paresthesia, a prickly and burning sensation in the hands or feet. Not overly common but just be aware.

3. Vitamin B12 – common in developing nations. Symptoms: a deterioration of the spinal cord, brain damage, fatigue, irritability and depression. If extreme, then certainly supplements are in order.

4. Vitamin K deficiency – common in developing countries with half of newborn infants, causes uncontrolled bleeding, under developed faces and bones. Also typically found in alcoholics, bulimics, strict dieters, cystic fibrosis. I suggest eating green vegetables.

5. Vitamin B2 deficiency – causes malnutrition, in alcoholics: pink tongue, cracked lips, throat swelling, bloodshot eyes, and low red blood cell count.

6. Vitamin D deficiency – can cause rickets: muscles and bones become soft; happens with some kids who are housebound. Reminder: D is

required for calcium to be absorbed. Sitting in the sun for ten minutes a day and/or in food or supplements will help.

7. Vitamin C deficiency – can cause "scurvy": lethargy, skin spots, bleeding gums, loss of teeth, fever and, in the extreme, death.

8. Vitamin B7 (biotin) – causes rashes, hair loss, anemia, drowsiness, and depression. Today found mainly in half of pregnant women, due to higher usage of it in the body.
Remedy: vitamin supplements

9. Vitamin B3 (niacin) – can cause Pellagra: symptoms are diarrhea, dermatitis, dementia, death. If you eat a variety of food in your diet it won't be a problem.

10. Vitamin B1 deficiency – can cause Beriberi, weight loss, bodily weakness, brain damage, irregular heart rate, heart failure and death. Found mainly in alcoholics whose bodies are poor in absorbing it.

Again, it is necessary to maintain a balanced immune system in every aspect. A periodic red blood analysis will render more certainty if you think you might be deficient in vitamins, along with a regular blood pane.

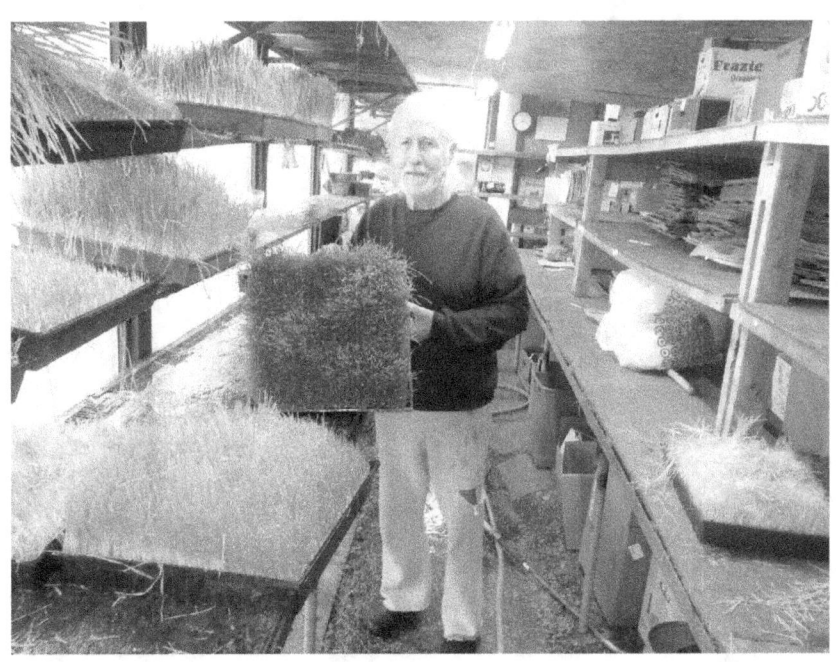

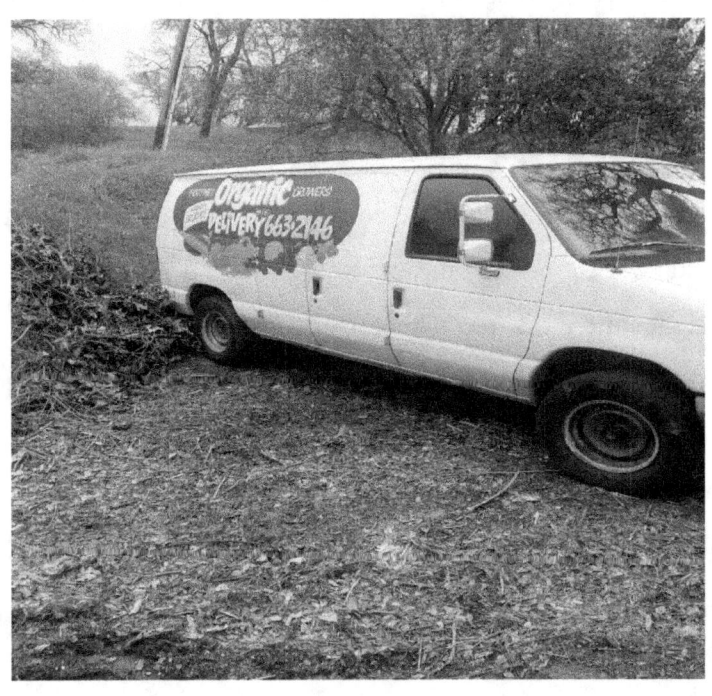

CH 17

THE MIRACLE OF WHEATGRASS
(Testimonial from a customer of "Organic Jack"--a California grower of Wheatgrass)

Lead words from Jack include the following: melanoma, fibromyalgia, nosebleeds, autism, mental clarity, energy, chronic pain, healthier skin, feeling better, shrinks tumors.

Dear Jack,

I want to take this time to write and thank you for your wonderful produce and your service to our community. As a person who has preached about and utilized the benefits of wheatgrass for much of my life to help others, I needed little convincing that this was the medicine my body needed. What I did need, though, was a knowledgeable person like yourself and come into my life and teach me.

When I called you in October, my ailments ranged from melanoma to fibromyalgia. I was suffering from sudden, chronic and very severe nosebleeds--which was indicative something even worse that was going on in my body. As you know I am the single mother of a special needs child (autism). My days are nonstop and I wasn't taking good care of myself. When I called you, I spoke of the need for good nutrition for myself and my child.

When you came to my home you advised me what foods in my cupboards were good for me, and bad for us. I knew you advice to us wasn't just about money, and that caring from you was a turning point in my life. I appreciate your caring so much.

Originally I called you for Wheatgrass because I had used it years ago. I also then decided to buy a harvest basket of fruits and veggies. I was in for an unexpected delight.

I had never known the advantage of eating organic produce before speaking with you. After 3 months of eating your fruit, I could smell and tell the difference between the chemical spayed fruits at the supermarket and yours. I now only purchase my produce in farmers markets, not at the store.

I now encourage people to juice with the Miracle MJ550. It is a great quality and I got mix good tasting fruits with wheatgrass. Sometimes I freeze the mix with a juice or 7up, and eat the nutritious ice cubes. For some parents who have children who are picky, this is a sure way they get their veggies and fruits.

In addition to having greater mental clarity, energy and reduction of pain in my body, I have healthier skin, and feeling better. How I treated and overcame the melanoma on my arms, I poured the wheatgrass juice on my arms, and gradually the cancer spots disappeared.

I have treated my dog's tumor on his leg in a similar and it worked. It disappeared on the spot. I believe too often we rely on our MDs to cure, and then they give us medicine which does not heal us, instead sometimes prolonging our healing. Wheatgrass is one of the most nutrient filled foods on the planet, and most importantly, it is SAFE for adults and children. Certainly it is the least costly medicine you can buy. $1.68/one box.

I also took my son off the Risperdal meds, an antipsychotic, prescribed by his doctor for autism. My son was having very frightening episodes of seizures, and was complaining of pain in his eyes. I researched this med and discovered it is not even approved by the FDA, yet it is prescribed for kids every day! My son's major symptoms have disappeared. And so I warn everyone, be sure to educate yourelf before taking any Pharm prescription. There is no doubt in my mind that if I had not taken my son off the med and used wheatgrass and organic foods, the end result would have been detrimental to him and me.

Thanks again, Jack I look forward to learning and sharing with you, as I work toward bringing myself and my family to optimum health.

Many blessings,
Polly Johnson

NOTE: Above is a photo of Jack inside his nursery this winter. He has a delivery service to customers who live in
towns and cities nearby. I have used his Wheatgrass as a
part of my cancer recovery. It possesses most of the vitamins and minerals and amino acids we all need to be healthy.

THANKS JACK – KEEP UP THE GREAT WORK!

CH 18

NEW HOPE UNLIMITED (Located in Arizona and Mexico)

I recently discovered this unique team of medical doctors dedicated to providing the most comprehensive treatment of chronic degenerative diseases and immune disorders, including cancers. Each of their members has been touched by illnesses of family members, or themselves personally. That is why they are developing progressive new treatment strategies that focus on the health of the body as well as the emotional and spiritual well-being of the patient and their family members.

The New Hope Unlimited cancer treatment program is designed with a personal approach to treating patients, offering a warm and caring atmosphere where every staff member focuses on the individual needs of the patient. Their major focuses are BUILDING THE IMMUNE SYSTEM, implementing anti-tumor protocols, and detoxification. There is a de-emphasis on chemo and radiation, and an emphasis on keeping the patient in remission with nutrition and with no recurrence of the cancer.

The medical staff at New Hope Alternative Cancer Center, therefore, focuses on restoring the powerful immune system with therapies such as the following:

*intravenous beet derived from levo-rotary vitamin C, which has been shown to increase immune cell activity, block carcinogens in the body, help in the elimination of virus infected cells, kill cancer cells, protect DNA from mutation, help eliminate carcinogens by increasing glutathione, and reduce pain.

*Treat hormone deficiencies in the body. DHEA, Melatonin, Thyroid and Thymus hormones provide powerful support.

*They also address the "internal Milieu" of the body, or connective tissue, or extra cellular fluid making up 50% of the body. As they point out the lifestyle of eating in this country has created an acidic condition, reduced oxygen levels decreased cellular nutrient intake and waste disposal, and the buildup of chemical toxins like pesticides and heavy metals like mercury, lead, cadmium, and arsenic. Cancer, like most other diseases, is a symptom of connective tissue and extra-cellular fluid/space degeneration.

*Restore the proper balance and function of healthy intestinal organisms in the intestine. The digestive tract plays a huge role in maintaining a healthy immune system. It is about 20 feet in length with an immense surface area that supports about 5 pounds of bacteria and fungi, most of which are beneficial to your health. However many things in our lives such as antibiotics, dietary sweets and alcohol and stress cause this delicate ecology to be upset. Overgrowth of fungi, atypical bacteria, parasites, delayed onset food sensitivities, "leaky bowel syndrome", and impaired nutrient assimilation can disturb and create a corrupted immune system.

* Body detoxification therapies in order to remove chemical toxins mentioned earlier.

*Treating nutritional deficiencies through proper diet and food supplements. One example as a common deficiency in the U.S.is 68% of us get less than two thirds of the recommended daily allowance. In my own case, as an older man, I discovered in my red blood cell analysis I was very deficient in vitamin B12. In essence, one cannot fight a cancer disease with a poor diet.

*The staff at the Center strongly believe the psychological and stress a person has undergone in his life can be contributory in their cancer diagnosis. They have realized the mind and the body are intimately connected. "Most of our patients recall events in their lives that disturbed them to the extent that they haven't been the same since." Many patients hold onto their anger, fears, sorrow, and eventually realizing "I can't take it anymore." The staff addresses these sorts of issues with a patient and considers it essential to their recovery process. The goal here is to reduce the pain with non-chemical means.

The total program addresses many more issues, specifically:

*live blood cell therapy
*oxygenating therapies
*colon therapies and enemas
*liver detox therapies
*Physical therapies and exercise
*Chiropractic to reduce pain

*Dental care

*Acupuncture-an Eastern approach which is 5,000 years old

*Ozone therapy- cancer cannot survive in an oxygen environment.

*Hyperbaric oxygen Chamber therapy

*Ultra violet blood irradiation therapy known to shrink large tumors.

I, in my own cancer treatment for my Melanoma in the lymph, used many of these therapies in my treatments. Obviously I survived so I know they can work if implemented by skilled practitioners.

Initially they have the patient stay in their Arizona facility for 12 days, for both treatments and education. Some are sent to Mexico, if it is necessary for their situation. Much of this information is online at their website.

CH 19

A HEALING TOUCH COULD MAKE A DIFFERENCE

One complimentary source to assist the patient with cancer is an age Tibetan treatment called REIKI. In his book REIKI: A HEALING HAND, William Lee Rand best describes Reiki as an unseen energy flow through all living things which affects the quality of health. Occasionally I used this method when in pain, when I couldn't sleep, or when others close to me were in pain or discomfort. I was trained in the Dr. Usui method 15 years ago and though I have not used it professionally, I have performed it on a voluntary basis. Some people had referred to it as ULF (Universal Life Energy).

Rand refers to it as a technique for stress reduction that also promotes healing, allowing everyone to tap into an "unlimited supply" of life energy. At the turn of the 20th century Reiki was discovered by D. Mikao Usui, a Japanese Buddhist. It is easy to learn. It has successfully been taught to thousands of people of all ages and religions. A treatment can feel like a wonderful glowing, warmth that comes from the treater and flows through your body. It creates many beneficial effects including relaxation and a feeling of peace, security and well-being. Many have experienced miraculous effects and it has been used by some as an adjunct in their cancer treatment.

One of the best testimonials regarding Rand's book on Reiki is as follows: Rand writes a book which is both spiritual and practical. His references to the source of Reiki and the higher power, the need for compassion and its relationship to healing helps us to remember the real purpose of healing.

Rand has done research in Japan, learning from different masters, which gave him a broad understanding so that his research is based on facts and original information from Japan, and not on second hand information that has wandered from the original intent of Reiki. He also includes all the hand positions, utilized for both self and others---which are very important to implement Dr. Usui's form of treatment.

The book is one of the clearest and easy to understand books on Reiki that I have experienced. Again, I do not consider this treatment as the be all and end all for use in assisting cancer patients, but it is well worth while as a stress and worry reducer. Having used it to reduce my pain, I suggest it in your choices of relief.

BENEFITS I RECEIVED FROM REIKI WHEN IN PAIN

About 14 years ago my back and left shoulder were in such pain that I could no longer get any relief from medications, plus I don't like putting foreign chemicals into my body. I met Karen, a Reiki Master. She explained the history and potential advantages which I might derive from treatments. I went to her for 3 treatments, each time she invoked her hand sign, a symbol for triggering life's energies. I felt a warm, relaxing feeling each time, the pain lessened but did not go away immediately.

On the 6th treatment it was mind-blowing! I could feel a deeper heat and a soothing of the muscles for about 10 minutes. Afterwards the pain was gone, and never returned. I became such a believer I decided to join a class, where eventually I learned to practice Reiki on others, using the hand formation and words to bring in this Life Energy. I don't practice Reiki professionally, however I had done it with relatives and friends. You can also use it on oneself, with high anxiety to calm down, and to help go to sleep at night.

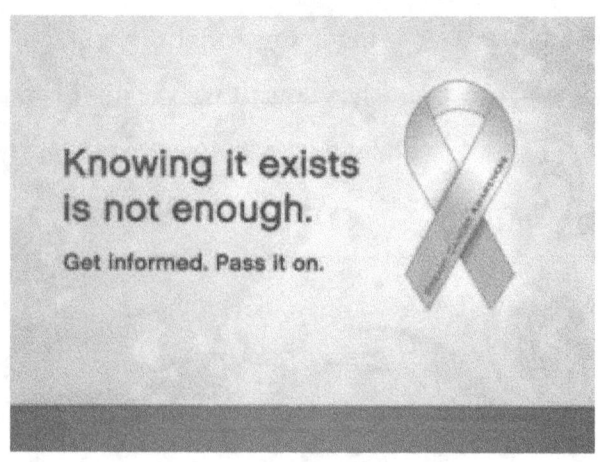

Knowing it exists
is not enough.

Get informed. Pass it on.

CH 20
CANCER MYTHS SCARING YOU?
NO NEED TO BE IN FEAR

Here I have compiled some of the more common myths which many people have erroneously accepted as fact when, in truth, they are inaccurate. The goal here is to learn the facts, plus some new ways to address the problem presented.

MYTHS FROM THE SKIN CANCER FOUNDATION

1. Eighty percent of a person's lifetime sun exposure is acquired before age 18, so if I am older it doesn't matter how much sun I get.
Fact: Only about 23% of lifetime exposure is acquired before age 18, so when one is older they should follow the best guidelines to avoid over exposure.

2. Tanning a salon is safer than tanning outdoors—it's a controlled dose of UV radiation.

Fact: Indoor tanners are at high risk for cancer. Frequent tanners receive high doses of UVA, sometimes 12X the dose of the sun's rays.

3. Some ingredients in sunscreen can cause cancer.

Fact: When used as directed it is not harmful. However, as an important part of protection, it is recommended to use SPF 15 or higher when in the sun.

4. The sun is the best way to get vitamin D.

Fact: Recommended: no more than 5 minutes in the sun at midday. Further UBV exposure damages the DNA in skin and breaks down vitamin D into ineffective pieces.

5. You can't get sun damage on a cloudy day.

Fact: Yes, you can. Up to 80% of the sun's rays penetrate clouds and fog. So bring out your protection of those days. Note: I got some of the worst burns in Santa Cruz, CA as a teenager on heavy fog days.

6. A "base tan" protects your body from sunburn.

Fact: There is no such thing as a safe tan. A tan is a sign of DNA sun damage. A tan is the body's way of repairing the damage.

7. I use a sun screen of SPF 50, so I'm all set.

Fact: Not entirely true. Most sun screens protect against UBV rays, but you need protection against UVB rays too.

Recommend: You need a broad spectrum (UVA/UVB) sunscreen for full protection.

8. People of color don't get skin color.
Fact: Not so, they may not get the types of cancer white folks get, but there is a rare type they must get checked for. Therefore they need protection and regular exams.

9. Windows protect us from the sun's ultra violet rays.
Fact: Glass inside a car blocks UVB rays, UVA can get through. So whether you're inside a house or in a car, you can get burns through glass. Suggestion: Buy window film to protect you.

NATIONAL CANCER INSTITUTE
Common Cancer Myths and Misconceptions

1. Cancer is like a death sentence.
Fact: Not necessarily so. How long an individual cancer patient will live depends upon many factors: is cancer slow of fast growing, how extensive the cancer has grown, whether effective treatments are available, the person's overall health, and more.

2. Will eating sugar make my cancer worse?
Fact: No. Although cancer research has shown cancer cells consume more sugar (glucose) than normal cells. No studies have shown eating sugar will make your cancer worse. However, a high sugar diet may contribute to excess weight gain, and obesity is associated with high risk of developing several types of cancer.

3. Artificial sweeteners cause cancer?

Fact: No. Researchers have conducted studies on the safety of sweeteners, such as saccharin (sweet low), aspartame (equal), NutraSweet, sucralose (Splenda)--all approved by the FDA.

4. Cancer is contagious.

Fact: In general, no. The only way it could spread is in the case of organ or tissue transplantation. Doctors avoid the use of tissues or organs from donors who have a history of cancer. In some people cancers may be caused by viruses, or HPV and bacteria Helicobacter pylori). They do not carry cancer when given to another.

5. My attitude can determine my risk for cancer.

Fact: To date, there is no convincing or scientific evidence that links a person's "attitude" to his risk of developing or dying from cancer. If you have cancer it is normal to have anger, sadness or discouraged. People with positive attitude may be more likely to have social connections and stay active, and activity and social support may help you to cope with your cancer.

6. Can cancer surgery or a tumor biopsy cause cancer to spread in the body?

Fact: Doubtful, the chance it will spread to other parts is extremely low. Surgeons take special steps to prevent spreading doing biopsies or surgery. For more information, see the NCI fact sheet on Metastatic Cancer.

7. Are there herbal products that can cure cancer?

Fact: No. Although some studies suggest herbs may help patients cope with side effects of cancer treatment.

Note: This statement is made from an Allopathic point of view and may not be accurate. It is recommended you study on topics of Complementary and Alternative Therapies regarding Botanicals/herbals that have been studied.

(This was only a partial list of myths)

CH 21
WHAT YOU NEED TO KNOW ABOUT L-GLUTATHIONE (GSH)

GSH is a powerful antioxidant and detoxifier, which can be found in every cell in our bodies. In a normal healthy body, sufficient levels of Glutathione can be found and this helps our immune system (among other things). L-Cysteine, L-Glutamic acid, and Glycine are able to synthesize this substance in our bodies, so it should not be necessary to introduce it in the food we eat.

However, as a result of the aging process and some chronic illnesses, levels of Glutathione can fall and this can increase our chances of attracting further problems. Unfortunately, increasing the body's level of Glutathione is not always easy, as much of the substance gets lost in the digestive system (when included in food), and the small amount that does get through is insufficient.

The most efficient way is to add this is intravenously, although using a liposomal delivery system is proving to be successful and almost as good as the former way.

Raising glutathione levels is also achieved by using drugs and natural products; these are usually called precursors or building blocks. One such precursor is N-acety-cysteine which is usually used to treat liver failure as a result of acetaminophen overdose. It has a short half-life and needs to be taken twice a day.

Glutathione is probably the most important antioxidant that the cells of our body produce, helping to neutralize oxygen compounds and free radicals. It can also regulate an essential cycle – the nitric oxide cycle – which is very important and vital for life, but can cause problems if not regulated correctly.

Glutathione has a direct effect on detoxifying foreign compounds and carcinogens, including heavy metals like lead and mercury. It also plays a big role in many metabolic and biochemical reactions. It is difficult to explain the exact functions of Glutathione without including a great deal of technical information, but even some doctors may find this difficult to understand unless they specialize in this particular area of medicine.

Basically, glutathione is considered to be the main antioxidant in our bodies, and a substance we cannot live without. It has the ability to attach itself to toxic chemicals in the liver and prepare them for elimination and removal from the body. These toxic chemicals include carbon monoxide, pesticides and heavy metals like mercury, lead, chromium and cadmium. It has also been suggested that glutathione might be able to control certain cancers, diabetes and other degenerative conditions.

Other areas that might benefit from glutathione are the treatment of hepatitis, cirrhosis and other liver diseases. Some asthmatic and pulmonary conditions have shown improvement by adding glutathione supplements to restore more normal levels.

CH 22
A NUTRITION TEST FOR YOUR BODY

I will list just ten of the items I learned about since being diagnosed with cancer 5 years ago. How many Americans have learned of these, including M.D.s in their practice? It is because the use of these foods and supplements that I was kept alive:

1. The best antioxidants.
2. The preferred waters to drink, to keep the body alkalized, and how to test for pH level in the blood as a guide to your health.
3. Enzyme supplements to assure dead cancer cells and other debris are flushed from the cells.
4. The importance of Thyroid gland supplements.
5. The importance of Adrenal gland functioning.
6. About the quality of the vitamins one is taking, for example, what are the better manufacturers?
7. Liver formulas to help detoxify a poisoned liver (especially important for anyone with any kind of life threatening disease.
8. What are the best Maca formulas which are major oxidants?
9. Have you read or heard of Life Extension Magazine which prints the best results foods and supplements for cancers? A great resource.
10. Have you had a live red blood cell analysis by a skilled doctor, to show you the state of your present blood condition? It can be done in a

physician's office and you can see the results of the formation of the cells on the computer screen. Afterwards, you will be instructed on what vitamins, herbs, or foods can improve your health.

I have this done every 3 months in order to satisfy myself that I am not deficient in any foods. Most hospitals and M.D.s do not offer this for their patients! Why not?

One of my main concerns here is to ask: Why are the family physicians and Oncologists not offering these vital pieces of information for the cancer patients? After all, knowing this material is what has saved my life and the lives of many thousands of people.

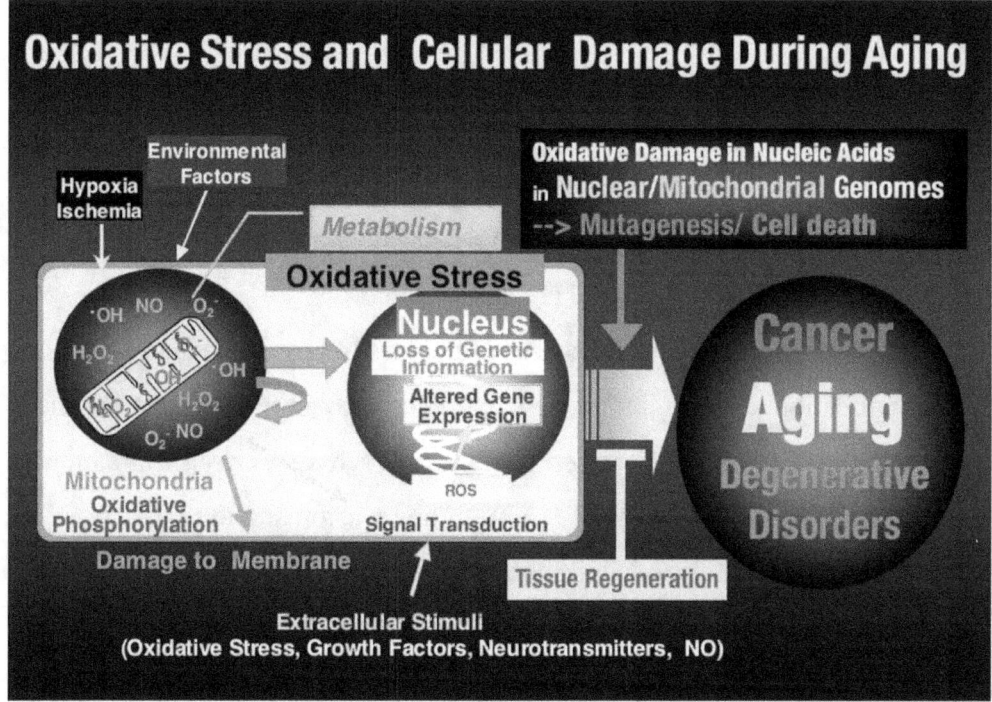

Oxidative Stress and Cellular Damage During Aging

CH 23
EFFECTS OF OXIDATION AND INFLAMMATION ON CANCER

Oxidation is a normal chemical reaction that occurs when free radicals form within the cells of an organism. Each oxygen atom contains two electrons that cling together. When heat or light breaks apart the atom, the electrons are separated, leaving unpaired oxygen radicals. These radicals are free to roam around, and initiate a process of breaking down normal cellular structures, causing damage and promoting the development of cancer. The more free radicals present, the more cancer causing damage.

The process is similar to what happens during the browning of an apple after it is sliced open and the flesh of the apple is exposed to the air. The oxygen atoms in the air interact with the sugar in the apple forming oxygen radicals. These radicals break down the flesh of the apple, or oxidize it, and the apple begins to rot. As long as the outer peel of the apple protects the inner flesh from oxygen, it is not oxidized.

The parallel in our bodies is when our tissues or organs are not protected with antioxidants or its own inner defenses against oxidation, then cancerous cells form and are allowed to grow.

One of the most common causes of the loss of protective antioxidants is inflammation, a biological process that your body initiates when fighting off an infection. If the body senses invaders such as bacteria, white blood cells are mobilized to go to the sight of the invasion and to release oxygen and nitrogen radicals to help kill their invaders. Sad to say, if they remain unchecked, these same oxygen radicals can also break down normal tissue, triggering cancer to develop. Oxygen radicals damage normal DNA, causing errors, allowing cancer growth.

With prostate cancer researchers have observed the presence of inflammatory cells in virtually all that tissue removed surgically and found that inflammation leads to atrophy, or wasting away, of normal prostate tissue adjacent to the precancerous and cancerous areas of prostate tissue.

Based on these observations, evidence shows that INFLAMMATION and OXIDATION play key roles in the development of prostate cancer. Yes, there other contributory factors such as aging and altered hormone secretions, however fundamental nutritional and exercise habits can be utilized to reduce these two factors.

Note: By including fresh fruits and vegetable in your diet, ocean caught fish, and whole grains, you can increase the anti-inflammatory parts of your diet. For example, tomato-based products such as soups, past and juices can increase levels of the antioxidant lycopene in the prostate gland. Drinking pomegranate juice and green tea can increase levels of antioxidant-containing polyphenols. Likewise, eating Broccoli, brussel sprouts, bokchoy, wasabi mustard, and horseradish can induce protective proteins in your liver and tissues, while vitamins, minerals, extracts of fruits and vegetables, herbs and spices can all act against oxidation land inflammation.

ZYMESSENCE: THE NEW BREED OF SYSTEMIC ENZYME BLENDS

William Wong, ND, PhD, member of the World Sports Medicine Hall of Fame teaches the applications of systemic enzymes: "Systemic enzymes are the most important part of maintaining a healthy body; of fighting the processes of aging and disease; and of undoing the planned obsolescence nature has built into our bodies to make sure we don't stay on the planet too long."

Systemic enzymes are the only non-toxic way of controlling inflammation of every type and from whatever reason. In fact they are the only tools available in both allopathic and naturopathic medicine for fighting fibrosis. Most of what ends up killing man is either an inflammation such as heart and vascular disease, diabetes, cancer, trauma, Alzheimer's, or a fibrosis related event such as a clot caused stroke or heart attack, fibrosis of the kidney, liver or heart valves; age related shrinking of the internal organs, etc. Inflammation is the #1 thing that brings about the formation of fibrosis and scar tissue. So control one and you prevent the formation of the other.

Dr. Wong originally discovered the German pharmaceutical labs were putting together the best enzymes in the world, top quality and, after a while, they developed not vegetarian enzymes but animal based ones which are much more potent, and they get the job done faster and more efficiently in the body. Instead of taking 30 pills a day with the former, the latter ones only need to be consumed 3- 6 capsules daily. He himself, with the help of a master Pharmacist, developed a product "Serrapeptase" which treats the following:

*Fibromyalgia
*Chronic fatigue
*Chronic pain or inflammation
*clogged arteries
*Fibroids
*Endometriosis
*Circulatory disorders
*Systemic yeast infections
*Autoimmune diseases
*post-operative scarring
*Fibrocystic breast disease
*Bladder infections

According to Dr. Wong, his product is a fast working systemic proteolytic enzyme on the planet with research to prove it. He asserts it works through every system in the body and organ preventing an accumulation of acidic waste, which bogs down the liver and the immune system function. I have been taking this product for several years, and believe it does work!

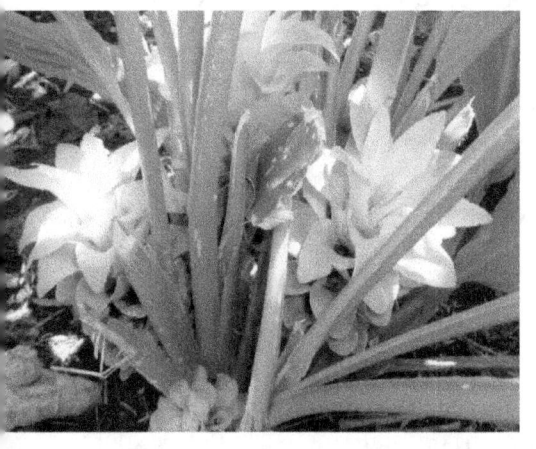
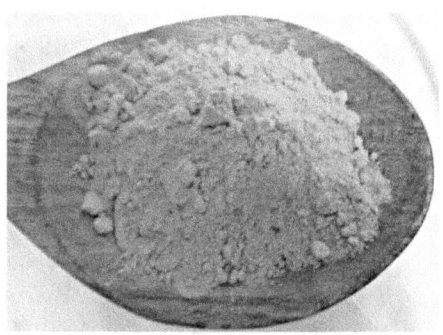

CH 24
TUMERIC—SPICES OF LIFE TO PREVENT CANCERS

This vegetable has an unbelievable history and healing effects and yet most Americans don't realize how much it can enhance our health. Even if Tumeric is not in your spice rack, you've probably tasted it. It has a warm, spicy taste and is found mostly in Middle Eastern dishes. It's the spice that colors and lends its scent to many kinds of mustard and gives them a distinctive, vibrant golden-yellow hue. It's also a principal ingredient in Worcestershire sauce and is used in jellies, relishes, cheeses, seasoning blends and more. It also compliments chili powder, coriander, cumin and cinnamon. It is also natural preservative.

It is the root of a tropical perennial known to botanists as Circuma longa, a member of the ginger family. It is native to China but also grows in the tropical regions of India and South America. India produces 90 percent of the world's supply of turmeric and is the largest producer.

Circumin is the major ingredient in Tumeric, with a remarkable range of therapeutic effects, including potent antitumor, antioxidant and anti-inflammatory properties. It has been used as an Ayurvedic medicine for 5,000 years. Unlike conventional Western medicine, Ayurvedic medicine does not draw sharp distinctions between food and medicine. Overall diet and specific foods are vital aspects of their therapies, and herbs, plants, oils and spices (especially Tumeric) are part of the Ayurvedic pharmacopeia.

They also use Tumeric to relieve pain, regulate menstruation, expel phlem, aid digestion and support healthy liver function. For people with colds and coughs and congestion, inhaling the fumes of burning turmeric may stimulate the flow of mucus and immediately relieve congestion.

How effective is Circumin with cancers? It has been used as an anti-inflammatory agent in many diseases and some cancers, and is known for its safety. Researchers at Baylor University Medical Center in Texas wrote in the Feb 2008 issue of Biochemical Pharmacology "that a spice once relegated to the kitchen shelves has moved in to the clinic and may prove to be "curecumin." Past trials indicate a potential therapeutic role for curecumin in diseases such as IBD, ulcerative colitis, colon cancer, pancreatic cancer, atherosclerosis, pancreatitis, psoriasis, and arthritis.

If, after the completion of many clinical trials currently underway in the U.S., Europe and Asia, circumin proves to be as effective as preliminary research suggests, it will not be the first time a naturally occurring substance becomes a therapeutic agent. Aspirin was derived from willowbark and Digitalis is made from the leaves of the foxglove plant.

One of the most exciting findings about circumin is its potential to prevent and treat various forms of cancer. Carcinogenesis, the development of cancer, involves three stages: initiation, progression and promotion. Circumin appears to inhibit all three of them, namely the inhibition of NF-kB and subsequent inhibition of pro inflammatory pathways as well as its ability to prevent the growth of new blood vessels. Circumin also has potential as a chemo protective agent, especially in the role of preventing colon cancer. Researchers at the University of Texas Medical Branch found Circumin blocked the activity of neurotensin, a hormone involved in the development of colon cancer.

Curcumin's potent antioxidant action protects cells from the free radicals that can harm cellular DNA. Thus it is most important in cells that undergo frequent turnover, such as those that line the digestive tract, because when these cells become cancerous they can reproduce quickly. Circumin has also been shown to inhibit the proliferation of some tumor cells in cell cultures, to prevent carcinogenic induced cancers in rodents. There are many examples of research done around the world to show the effects of Circumin on inhibiting many different cancers, too many to mention herein. Some top medical researchers are excited about results they are observing because Circumin is inexpensive and is very safe to administer, with no side effects.

Again be sure to consult with your Holistic or Naturopathic doctor before and during use. I am not suggesting this is the only treatment for colon cancer, but is certainly worth your consideration.

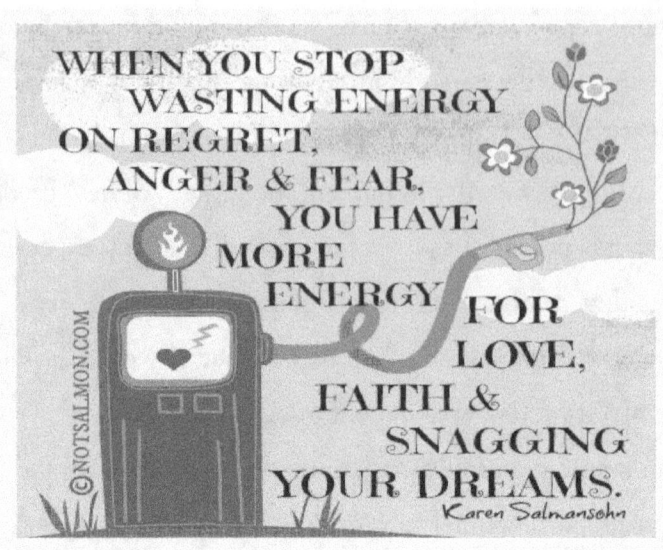

WHEN YOU STOP WASTING ENERGY ON REGRET, ANGER & FEAR, YOU HAVE MORE ENERGY FOR LOVE, FAITH & SNAGGING YOUR DREAMS.
Karen Salmansohn
©NOTSALMON.COM

CH 25
ANGER, DOUBT, AND FEAR WILL NOT SERVE YOU WELL
A negative emotional response to your cancer could prevent healing

It is true. If you don't quickly shift beyond your initial reaction to hearing you have cancer in your body, things could get worse. Most people I have met who recovered from their cancer have shared with me: To not gain a proper perspective could bring about more pain, a worsening of your treatment, more conflicted relationships with your relatives and friends and, possibly, hasten an even earlier death. I can, as a cancer survivor, relate to those feelings.

When the Oncologist surgeon informed my relatives in the lobby of the hospital after the surgery--he had located 10 metastasized tumors under my left arm--he informed them the odds of recovery were poor. As I was awakening from the surgery and certain relatives approached, I saw the caution in their eyes and the inflection of their voices; they did not believe

I would recover. I, at that time was in denial. After all I was healthy most of my life, and didn't think of myself as a sick guy.

A week later was a different feeling for me. My doctor let me know that those with Melanoma have it in the entire lymphatic system, and most do not survive longer than 3-6 months. I accepted the fact he had no options for a cure for me. And he admitted his total ignorance of any nutritional supplements with which to rebuild the immune system. It was time for me to take independent action, so I sought out a Naturopath who knows about healing herbs, since I had met a 74 year old man who was dying of severe heart and lung complications who had extended his life 7 years. His doctor, who previously did not believe in herbs for health suddenly became a believer when he saw how my friend recover and extend his life. My friend convinced me to take herbs for good health and so I did not forget his words.

Moreover, armed with his testimonial to me, I decided to go to Sunrise Natural Foods in Roseville, Ca. and find a knowledgeable worker. I then met Alden Okie, who had advised others for 15 years about herbs and natural foods. He shared he had suffered from a chronic immune deficiency disease. His doctor informed him he was a hopeless case and would die soon. Nine years later, with proper herb and food intake, Alden shared he is in perfect health and energy, with normal blood readings now. He then gave me some essential facts on the immune system. At last I started feeling somewhat hopeful.

He then referred me to Dr. Ward Joiner, DC, HNT, a Holistic doctor here in Roseville, CA. I gained an immediate appointment with Joiner: He shared his own personal history of very poor health as a child, as an adult and his road to recovery. He was weak as a child, developed multiple diagnoses with various illnesses: lupus, immune deficiencies, chronic fatigue, etc. In his 40s, his doctor felt he would die soon and should shut down his private practice. He did and was disabled for six years. The good news: He chose to adopt a nutritional protocol which wiped out his infections, and today he is well, working 12 hours a day, helping others with life threatening problems. Inspired by the stories of these two men, I decided to hire Dr. Joiner to guide my path to recovery.

Dr. Joiner was very specific with me: "I don't cure cancer; the body can do that if it is fed correct foods." He recommended only natural foods and supplements, and no pharmaceutical manufactured products "because the body will not recognize them for its well-being."

HAVE YOU NOTICED ALL THE HORRIBLE POSSIBLE SIDE EFFECTS FROM THE DRUGS BEING ADVERTISED ON TV LATELY?

Dr. Joiner derived from my blood analysis results I was low-low in Testosterone, T-cells, NK cells, and IGF-1 proteins. He told me weeks later: "you were almost dead when you first walked in my office."

Psychologically and emotionally, from the very first day I met him, I knew I would not have to suffer from my cancer, even though I might someday die from it. He felt by improving my immune system, my body might be able to fight off the cancer cells gradually. Over the months he did more blood readings, and each time I felt more optimistic as my energy level improved. Indeed I slept better every night thereafter, just knowing we were on the right track to health.

MY OWN PSYCHOLOGY OF HEALING

As a trained family Therapist in California, in addition to my own personal life experiences, I had always wished for whole health for my clients, and for myself. I sought not partial healing, but complete healing. Why? Because partial healing meant I would be in psychic pain along with some physical pain. "No thanks" I said to myself when cancer appeared.

I am not an advocate for choosing methods of recovery which might induce pain and suffering. I am anti-suffering for both myself and my clients. So I said to myself: "Self, you could try the conventional way of attacking cancer with chemo, radiation, or interferon – all of which will lower the immune systems chances for survival – and cause suffering; or choose a nutritional approach with zero side effects, in order to power up the immune system (the only real way to defeat cancer cells). Dr. Joiner used an interesting imagery for me to consider: "Cancer is the enemy, remember the Pac-Man game on computers; we want to shoot them down one at a time."

Furthermore, my attitude before my diagnosis was, and still is, if good nutrition worked so well for others in their illnesses and they survived, it just might work for me. I knew the Melanocytes would attack me and kill me in a few months; therefore I could not wait another year for the Allopathic or conventional doctors to do their long term longitudinal studies to invent a cure. Through my own research I sensed the narrow, tunnel vision approach of the Allopathics, often motivated by greed and power, would not serve me well. I chose the Naturopathic way, knowing I'd have a chance to live longer and/or die with minimal suffering.

I rejected pharmaceutical pill, injections and began to avoid all food products which would destroy my immune system. Why? Because clearly the medical profession as a whole admits they do not have a cure for cancers. In reality, only the body's own chemistry can balance and heal itself.

My emotional state today, 5 years since my diagnosis, is free, peaceful and confident that I made the right decisions. In that respect, I still feel responsible for my outcomes. There will be no one to blame if my plan backfires. True responsibility is a no blame state of being. It is clean, with fresh air. It is freedom at its best. The best words for my journey now are that IT IS STILL A REAL CHALLENGE, AND SO FAR I AM WINNING, going on 5 years since my surgery.

It is also an honor to share my victory with other cancer patients who are having doubts about their possible treatments of choice. If you were recently diagnosed with cancer, keep an open mind. Perhaps, too, you might choose a combination of conventional treatments along with some natural food products. I have heard some medical doctors say that Naturopathic doctors are "quacks." My perception is just the opposite: the MDs appear to be the real quacking ducks, using their tortuous methods on cancer patients, with little or no hope of recovery, and with a painful process leading up to death by the end of the 5th year. Until they are willing to adopt an INTEGRATED MODEL OF CANCER TREATMENT, which includes educating themselves about the great value of nutritional remedies, they are not to be trusted. There are a few doctors who grasp this need to expand and develop complementary and alternative treatments, but they are the exception at this time.

In summary, it is little wonder the death statistics annually for cancer patients are the evidence the present systems of treatment have failed. Please don't just believe me. Do you research and draw your own conclusions. Remember I recovered from a potentially fatal disease with Melanoma phase IV, and thank God I did not trust the establishment.

CH 26
TESTIMONIALS FROM CANCER PATIENTS AND RECOMMENDED BOOKS

One of the persons Suzanne Somers interviewed for her book "Knockout" was Bill Falloon, founder of Life Extension, Inc., when he said: "The second biggest killer in America is medical ignorance and it is the no.1 reason people die." He enumerated, as an example, if you choose the conventional treatment for cancer, cutting, chemotherapy, or radiation, doctors are refusing to:

1. Choose nontoxic approaches to treating cancer
2. Recognize that after surgery there is higher risk of cancer spreading to other organs without a nutritional remedy
3. Sharing that surgery induces immune suppression
4. Know it is important to boost a person's immune system before surgery--so that the cancer cells that escape during surgery are killed by active immune cells.

If one is electing surgery, what is there to consume in order to inhibit cancer cells adhesion to normal cells? It is Bill Falloon's contention what works are two things: a supplement modified citrus pectin. Second, Cimetidine, suppresses cancer cell adhesion, according to the British

Journal of Cancer 2002 edition. In a study of Melanoma from a journal of the National Cancer Institute, Melanoma's were reduced by 90%!

The mystery to me is why Oncologists are refusing to use this well researched advice. I learned from an M.D. recently that most medical schools don't teach nutrition, or doctors only take one class before they graduate.

ABOVE ALL, I SUGGEST YOU SEEK TESTIMONIALS FROM THOSE WHO OVERCAME THEIR CANCER, AFTER BENG DIAGNOSED

Phase 2-4 chances for recovery--by having eaten a healthy change of foods, waters, antioxidants, enzymes and herbal supplements. Contrary to what many Oncologist M.D.s might tell a patient, not only are Holistic Nutritionists not "quacks", but many patients have given positive, evidence-proven information on how they recovered by maintaining their alkalinity, eating the right foods, and avoiding acid producing foods.

These patients are willing to tell their stories of recovery and, the best part of their stories is that they did not suffer from the horrible side effects of chemo and radiation for weeks and months, nor die in the end.

In my own case, my story is best summarized in a flyer I prepared for Organic Jack of Newcastle, CA, the organic farmer with a heart and the knowledge to go with it. "I salute you, Jack! You have, along with Dr. Joiner, saved my life with a long bout of Melanoma in my lymph system. You convinced me to start juicing with Wheatgrass and I know this has been instrumental in my recovery from one of the most devastating cancers. According to my most recent P.E.T. scan (which can track malignancies), my body is now clear from all metastasized cancer cells. Allelulia!"

Yes, I do use other products, herbal foods, antioxidantfruits and veggie greens. I also take Dr. Joiner's recommended protocol of amino acids, vegetable enzymes, Adrenal supplements, Thymic gland formula, etc.to strengthen my immune system.

Lastly, Wheatgrass enabled my blood system to remain alkalized. Just recently I learned babies, born healthy, possess healthy immune systems which are alkalized--and cancers cannot survive in alkalized state. They prefer an acidic state.

Another testimonial: C.C., a middle aged woman recovered from "terminal" Glioblastoma Multiforme (GBM IV brain tumor) diagnosis. Her PhD Nutritionist placed her on an intensive protocol of diet,nutritional schedule as follows: reduce sugar intake, Siberia Ginseng, astralagus, cat's claw and mushroom extracts. Next she took 16 IP6 capsules, along with genestein, bromelain, berberine,glutathione, quercetin,and proanthocyandidins. (I have taken some of these supplements myself) The patient also chose to refuse chemotherapy from her doctor; instead chose radiation. She followed the recommendation of her. Nutritionist before and after the surgery, suffered no side effects as a result. The MRI done afterwards revealed the tumor had responded well.

A third inspiring story comes from Lorraine Day, M.D., who in 1992 was diagnosed with StageIV Breast Cancer. She was chief of Orthopedic Surgery at San Francisco General Hospital, and for 15 years was on the faculty at U.C.S.F. School of Medicine. As a medical doctor she chose not to have chemotherapy, instead choosing "diet therapy" as her cancer recovery program. She stopped eating animal products, instead eating only fruits, greens and vegetables. As a result, she completely recovered. She did have a lumpectomy of a small tumor, but the tumor did recur, became aggressive and grew rapidly. Dr. Day rejected standard therapies because of their destructive effects and because these therapies often led to death. She chose instead to rebuild her immune system, using the natural, simple inexpensive foods designed by God--so that her body could heal itself. This, too, is my belief in my situation.

There are two videos of Dr.Day I suggest you see On Line: "You can't improve on God" and "Cancer doesn't scare me anymore."

SOURCES OF BOOKS, MAGAZINES, JOURNALS, TO FACILITATE YOUR CHOISE OF TREATMENT REMEDIES FOR HEALING YOUR IMMUNE SYSTEM

*Medical Journals
*Health magazines
*NCI Data base
*Internet authors and their books on cancer
*books on the pH factor
*AMA (American Medcal Association) resources
*cancerfightingstrategies.com (some of the best information on the internet
* My personal consultants:
Dr. Ward Joiner, DC, HNT myholistichealth.net
Organic Jack (provides me with Wheatgrass on a regular basis) Newcastle, CA. www.organicjack@sbcglobal.com

Some of my FAVORITE BOOKS:

*A RETURN TO HEALING - Len Saputo, M.D. describes his vision of the expansion of Integral Health Care Medicine serving cancer patients--better than anyone. I personally met and spoke with Dr. Saputo, a brilliant leader in the field. A very diversified healer of cancer patients, emphasizing assisting the patient to find best choices amongst available alternatives. This is a true five star rating author.

*WHAT ARE SYSTEMIC ENZYMES AND WHAT DO THEY DO?
Dr. Wm. Wong, PhD, ND, member World Sports Medicine Hall of Fame--recommends supplementing our cancerous bodies with the following:
--a natural anti-inflammatory
--anti-fibrosis (scar tissue)
--Blood cleansing, to breakdown dead material in the blood and cleanse the FC receptors on white blood cells--to help fight off infection

* "Knockout" by Suzanne Somers
She interviewed doctors who are successful in cancer recovery and immune builders, Nutritional protocol experts. An excellent book.

* "Cancer Recovery Guide": 15 Alternatives and Complementary Strategies for Restoring Health" by Jonathon Chamberlain

* "Outsmart Your Cancer" by Tanya Pierce

* Healing the Gerson Way" by Charlotte Gerson 441 pages, a large read but worth reading as a reference: a schedule for eating for cancer patients, describes coffee enemas as a way of detoxifying and purging the body of toxins. 60 complete recipes.

* "The Acid-Alkaline Food Guide" by Susan E. Brown, an easy toread guide to the common foods that influence the body's pH level.
An excellent guide for patients in preparing and cooking meals.
A short and inexpensive book.

* "How to Prevent and Treat Cancer with Natural Medicine" by Michael Murray – very lengthy but rich in alternative treatments. Besides diet, it mentions studies on acupuncture, hydrotherapy, and massage. Endorsed by the Cancer Treatment Center of America, authorized by 4 Naturopathic physicians. A good reference manual.

*www.pawpawresearch.com by Dr. Jerry McLaughlin--
Paw paw is an herb from a tree which, when processed and picked correctly, may be one of the best antioxidants. I take it still. He claims it actually can act synergistically with chemotherapy--making it more effective.

*LIFE EXTENSION MAGAZINE
Bill Falloon, Founder and Editor
This is the very best magazine in Holistic literature. Many M.D.s are listed who are involved in their own in house research and development of nutritional remedies and supplements, for many life

threatening diseases.

*THE IMMUNE SYSTEM RECOVERY
by Susan Blum, M.D. – emphasis on the Immune System giving the patient safe and natural ways to heal. Like myself, she sees food as the most fundamental and powerful mediator of health and wellness. She serves on the medical Advisory Board of the Dr. Oz TV show.

*CANCER: STEP OUTSIDE THE BOX"
by Ty M. Bollinger – shows proven strategies for avoiding surgeries, radiation or chemo. List some of the best nontoxic treatments in the world. Like myself and many others, he states the big Pharmas and many doctors are costing thousands of cancer patients their very lives. Definitely worth reading.

I have many more suggestions for readers. Feel free to call me and I will share some very effective quality products I have taken to overcome Melanoma. John W. Hall, Author 916-705-6624
Best time to call is 7-9 a.m. or evenings Pacific Time.

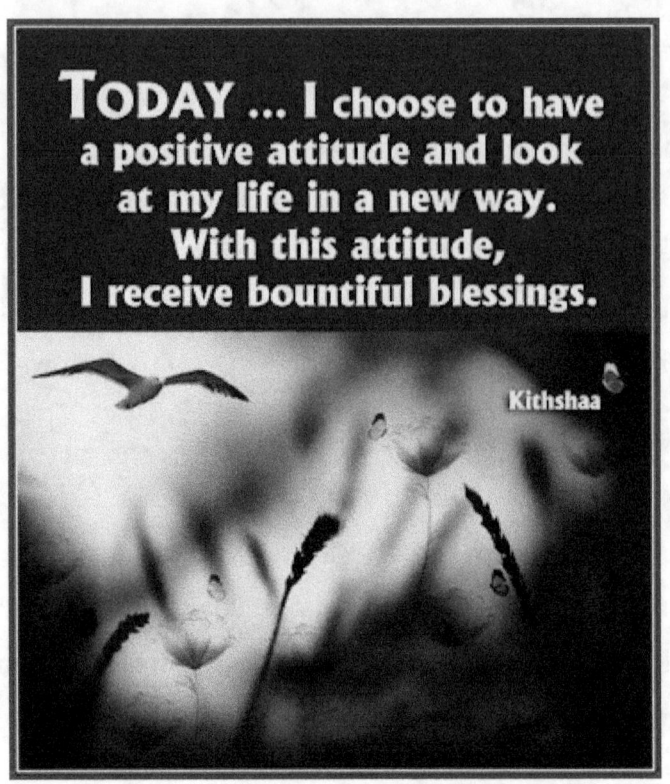

TODAY ... I choose to have a positive attitude and look at my life in a new way. With this attitude, I receive bountiful blessings.

Kithshaa

CH 27
IS THERE A GOD, HOLY SPIRIT, OR HIGHER POWER PROTECTING ME?
HE CREATED US, HE CAN HEAL US

My belief is: God gave us life. We don't know how He did it. He provided us with all the water, oxygen, trees, soils, and sun so that we could have healthy bodies on planet earth. He did not intend for us to suffer but rather the opposite, to thrive and have vibrant energy. He also gave us the brain power to correct things as they go wrong. Since age 7 I have believed He is all giving, all healing, all forgiving Spirit, an all-Loving Creator.

Many times in my life has he preserved me from early death: an auto accident at age 17 where the car crashed and I was thrown through the windshield. We had struck a high powered power pole at 65 mph. Results were I had severe cuts and bruising, and a head concussion with chronic headaches for 18 months. Then seven years ago doctors detected an Aortic Abdominal Aneurism, a bent blood vessel about to burst, and the doctor saved me from bleeding to death by inserting a Stent in the large blood vessel, which straightened it out. That was truly a lease on life.

We all have stories on how we were protected from birth and onward in life. There is a power bigger than us. Why? I don't know. What I do know is the Spirit-Creator is very generous with us, all giving. I believe He expects us to honor His creations, especially our own body. One last thought: If we are intentionally taking in foods that are poisonous, breathing in toxic substances such as smoke, cigarette smoke, living around radioactive stuff, eating GMOs, which might cause cancer or other life threatening diseases, then it seems we are dishonoring His plan.

My conclusions for eliminating my anger, doubt and fears around the subject of cancer are as follows:

1. Recognizing my body was provided with all the needed hormones, blood cells, tissues, and organs to cure it of invading pathogenic organisms.

2. Attitude: I was thankful to place my trust in God, for better or worse, and being appreciative of the modern diagnostic equipment, especially for the P.E.T. scan which enabled my Oncologist to identify the location of some of the malignant tumors.

3. I trusted the M.D. surgeon who helped me make the choice to have the surgery or not. I had 28 tumors, 10 metastasized, most removed in surgery.

4. I trusted my Holistic Nutritionist, Dr. Ward Joiner to become my coach. He recommended a protocol of amino acids, super vitamins, healthy foods, alkalized waters, greens, antioxidants, thymic gland formulas, Adrenal formulas and animal and veggie enzymes.

5. I took full responsibility, for better or worse, for my choice of an Allopathic doctor or a Naturopathic one.

6. Having gratitude to my Creator for his inspiration to lead me to making good decisions. One of my favorite quotes from the book "A Course in Miracles," says it the best: "...gratitude to God becomes the way to which He is remembered, for Love cannot be far behind a grateful heart and thankful mind." M55/58

7. Being thankful to all of you who supported me during my recovery.

8. I have eternal gratitude that I have resided in the U.S. where we have freedom of speech to elect a path to recovery.

9. I chose some affirmations to myself, to overcome my fears and anxieties:

"I am a creation of God and am worthy of good health."
"I value life with minimal or no pain or suffering, for myself and others."
"I am open to Holy Spirit to provide the guidance I need to conquer my cancers."

10. I daily ask for enlightenment from on High that this disease we call cancer will be eradicated from the planet soon.

My feelings are strong and with positive thoughts in spite of what I have been through. I realize the "hope pills" the Allopathic doctors and pharmas tried to sell me, and the "wishing you well" messages from well-meaning friends are not enough to overcome or manage my cancer. My recovery requires some research on my part, concentrating on sticking to a healthy eating program, and to my being open to any new, effective research results.

It is my intention to remain totally responsible to whatever the outcome with these Melanomas. I have already extended my life for five years with the help of many people – and it is my hope whoever reads this book and implements some of the ideas will achieve some of the positive results I am enjoying.

JOHN W. HALL, M.A., AUTHOR, CANCER SURVIVOR